DISABILITY JUSTICE IN PUBLIC HEALTH EMERGENCIES

Disability Justice in Public Health Emergencies is the first book to highlight contributions from critical disability scholarship to the fields of public health ethics and disaster ethics. It takes up such contributions with the aim of charting a path forward for clinicians, bioethicists, public health experts, and anyone involved in emergency planning to better care for disabled people—and thereby for all people—in the future. Across 11 chapters, the contributors detail how existing public health emergency responses have failed and still fail to address the multi-faceted needs of disabled people. They analyze complications in the context of epidemic and pandemic disease and emphasize that vulnerabilities imposed upon disabled people track and foster patterns of racial and class domination.

The central claim of the volume is that the ethical and political insights of disability theory and activism provide key resources for equitable disaster planning for all. The volume builds upon the existing efforts of disability communities to articulate emergency planning priorities and response measures that take into account the large body of qualitative and quantitative research on disabled people's health, needs, and experiences. It is only by listening to disabled people's voices that we will all fare better in future public health emergencies.

The book will be of interest to scholars and graduate students working in bioethics, disability studies, public health policy, medical sociology, and the medical humanities.

Joel Michael Reynolds is a Senior Research Scholar at the Kennedy Institute of Ethics, an Associate Professor of Philosophy and Disability Studies at Georgetown University, Faculty in the Pellegrino Center for Clinical Bioethics and the Department of Family Medicine at the Georgetown University School of Medicine and Medical Center, and a Senior Advisor to and Fellow of The Hastings Center. They are author or coauthor of six books and over sixty publications spanning philosophy, public health, and biomedical ethics.

Mercer E. Gary is an Assistant Professor of Philosophy at Drexel University and a Presidential Scholar at The Hastings Center. Her first book, *The Limits of Care: Making Feminist Sense of Technology Relations*, is under contract with Oxford University Press.

DISABILITY JUSTICE IN PUBLIC HEALTH EMERGENCIES

*Edited by Joel Michael Reynolds and
Mercer E. Gary*

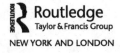

NEW YORK AND LONDON

Cover Image via Getty: Marcin Lukasiak

First published 2025
by Routledge
605 Third Avenue, New York, NY 10158

and by Routledge
4 Park Square, Milton Park, Abingdon, Oxon, OX14 4RN

Routledge is an imprint of the Taylor & Francis Group, an informa business

ISBN: 978-1-032-82035-4 (hbk)
ISBN: 978-1-032-82033-0 (pbk)
ISBN: 978-1-003-50262-3 (ebk)

DOI: 10.4324/9781003502623

Typeset in Times New Roman
by SPi Technologies India Pvt Ltd (Straive)

CONTENTS

List of Contributors   *vii*

Why Only Disability Justice Can Prepare Us for the Next
Public Health Emergency   1
Mercer E. Gary and Joel Michael Reynolds

PART I
Crisis in the Clinic   **15**

1 Disability Rights and Disability Justice as Gestalt Shifts for Triage
   Decision-Making in a Pandemic   17
   Katie Savin and Laura Guidry-Grimes

2 Incorporating Social Determinants of Health into Crisis Standards of Care 33
   April Dworetz

3 Tragic Choices: Disability, Triage, and Equity Amidst a Global Pandemic   47
   Joseph A. Stramondo

PART II
Multiply Marginalized   **57**

4 "We Are a Compromise": A Social Security Model of Disability
   During COVID-19   59
   Katie Savin

5 Chronic Injustice: Racialized Disablement and the Urgency of the Everyday 71
Desiree Valentine

6 Long COVID and Disability: Navigating the Future 84
Nicholas G. Evans

7 Patient-Centered Communication and Resource Allocation
for Non-Speaking People During Crises 95
Ally Peabody Smith

PART III
Before the Next Pandemic **105**

8 Long COVID and Disability Justice: Critiquing the Present, Forming
the Future 107
Sarah Clark Miller

9 Not Everything is a Pandemic: The Challenge of Disability Justice 120
Perry Zurn

10 Education as Bioethics: Oppression and Pandemic Public Education 135
Kevin Timpe

11 Building Institutional Trustworthiness in Emergency Conditions:
Lessons from Disability Scholarship and Activism 150
Corinne Lajoie

Index *164*

CONTRIBUTORS

April Dworetz Department of Pediatrics, Emory University, Atlanta, GA, USA

Nicholas G. Evans Department of Philosophy, University of Massachusetts Lowell, Lowell, MA, USA

Laura Guidry-Grimes Department of Medicine, Cleveland Clinic Lerner College of Medicine, Cleveland, OH, USA

Corinne Lajoie Faculty of Arts and Humanities, Western University, London, Ontario, Canada

Sarah Clark Miller Department of Philosophy, Pennsylvania State University, State College, PA, USA

Katie Savin Division of Social Work, California State University, Sacramento, CA, USA

Ally Peabody Smith College of Health, Lehigh University, Bethleham, PA, USA

Joseph A. Stramondo Department of Philosophy, San Diego State University, San Diego, CA, USA

Kevin Timpe Department of Philosophy, Calvin College, Rapids, MI, USA

Desiree Valentine Department of Philosophy, Marquette University, Milwaukee, WI, USA

Perry Zurn Department of Philosophy and Religion, American University, Washington, DC, USA

WHY ONLY DISABILITY JUSTICE CAN PREPARE US FOR THE NEXT PUBLIC HEALTH EMERGENCY

Mercer E. Gary and Joel Michael Reynolds

On January 30, 2020, the World Health Organization declared a *Public Health Emergency of International Concern* (PHEIC) over what would quickly become known as SARS-CoV-2 or COVID-19. This emergency status was officially ended in the United States in May 2023 amidst much dissent and debate. Although emergency conditions resulting from COVID-19 will likely wax and wane over the coming years, there is good reason to think that the incidence of severe global pandemics will increase over the next century, as will declarations of emergency (Curseu et al. 2009; The Lancet Planetary Health 2021). The declaration of an emergency calls for urgent action, but it just as urgently demands careful reflection. Official "emergency" status licenses unparalleled executive intervention, completely reorganizing the lives of those who live under its decree. Such official recognition, however, is heavily dependent on the social context in and from which the emergency arises. Highlighting *which* circumstances rise to the level of an official emergency clarifies our reigning assumptions about what threshold of active harm—and in relation to which groups of people—demands immediate intervention.

This volume articulates the contributions of critical disability scholarship for thinking about emergencies, especially in relation to research in bioethics and public health ethics. The essays collected here emerged from a symposium held virtually at Georgetown University in November 2021, driven by a sense of the urgent need for more critical disability perspectives in pandemic scholarship and response. Our central claim is not simply that existing public health emergency responses have failed and still fail to address the multifaceted needs of disabled people, but rather that the ethical and political insights of disability theory and advocacy provide key resources for equitable disaster planning for all. Anticipating arguments across the 11 chapters, we begin by reviewing the standards governing the declaration of a public health emergency as well as the practical and political implications of such a declaration. By examining these standards, we place in sharper relief the emergency conditions that lack official recognition. As the United States has now officially announced an "end" to this years-long public health emergency, we will also consider what the loss of this official status will mean for the provision of pandemic response resources.

DOI: 10.4324/9781003502623-1

The declaration of a public health emergency is an administrative rallying cry, one pitched to correspond to the severity of the present threat. Such threats are diverse, including infectious disease outbreaks, bioterrorist attacks, natural disasters, humanitarian crises, or other forms of disorder that pose an imminent threat to population health (see HHS, Sect. 319; WHO Emergencies Programme). Public health emergencies fall under the broader umbrella of disasters, which philosopher Naomi Zack has defined as "an event (or series of events) that harms or kills a significant number of people or otherwise severely impairs their daily lives in civil society" (Zack 2009, 6).[1] The World Health Organization's designation of a PHEIC emerged only in 2005, in the wake of the 2003 SARS-CoV epidemic. Since then, the WHO has declared six PHEICs, all of which were the result of disease outbreaks. Though not the only factors at play, virulence and spread carry considerable weight in such a declaration: fellow deadly coronavirus SARS-CoV saw 8,096 infections and 774 deaths at a rate of 9.6% while the 2012 MERS-CoV epidemic resulted in 2,553 infections and 876 deaths at a rate of 34.3% (Zhu et al. 2020). At the time of the January 2020 declaration, there were 7,818 confirmed cases and 2,977 deaths associated with COVID-19 across 19 countries and five WHO regions (WHO Novel Coronavirus Report). Unlike SARS-CoV and MERS-CoV, COVID-19's high viral shedding in the early stages of infection and proportion of asymptomatic or mildly symptomatic cases capable of transmitting the virus have made community spread particularly difficult to control (Wu et al. 2021).[2] These factors number among what Zack calls the "objective features" of a disaster.

But disease factors alone do not an emergency make. Rather, it is the "exigency, calamitous harm, [and] unavoidability of harm through ordinary processes" in combination with disease factors that legitimate the declaration of a public health emergency (Haffajee et al. 2014). The transformation of a viral threat into a full-fledged emergency for the public is therefore dependent on the social and political conditions into which the virus enters: factors like patterns and modes of travel, frequency of large public gatherings, housing availability, and reliability of access to food, water, and electricity number among the circumstantial determinants of an emergency. Absent conditions for substantial community transmission, even the most infectious disease would fail to meet the threshold of calamitous harm. Likewise, where ordinary processes are robust enough to respond effectively to an imposing threat, harms become avoidable and escalation interrupted. It stands to reason, then, that an unequal distribution of resources before a crisis begins will place some institutions in better positions than others to maintain normal functioning.[3] In other words, the onset of an emergency will be felt most acutely when and where the chips are already down.

On the other hand, we seem to be *less* likely to call an event a disaster or emergency if it occurs within patently unequal background conditions. Zack explains this apparent paradox by way of a distinction between disaster and risk: following widely held intuitions, Zack takes disasters to mark a significant departure from one's normal life. Where significant threats of harm have extended for long periods of time and have become sedimented within a particular social milieu, what in an acute crisis would be called a disaster is more appropriately described as a *risk* that can nonetheless be incorporated into normal daily life (Zack 2009, 4–6). Here Zack juxtaposes the threat posed by automobile accidents—which resulted in 6 million deaths globally between 2002 and 2007—and avian flu—which led to 192 deaths during the same period. The risk of traffic fatalities, though considerably higher than the risk of death by avian flu, does not pose the same kind of disruption to society precisely because they are so much more common (Zack 5). The familiarity of institutional procedures and social norms for handling automobile accidents, combined with societal dependence on cars for transportation and societal normalization of the deaths such transportation hastens, highlight the extent to which the risks of driving are treated neither as a disaster nor an emergency but as normal and ordinary within contemporary life.

The conversion of disaster into risk is not necessarily negative, given the unavoidability of danger and the practical utility of developing habituated responses to it. But it's also clear that this conversion process operates unevenly, enabling dominant groups to downgrade the urgency of events lived as emergencies by marginalized populations. When borne primarily by the underclasses, circumstances that meet the objective criteria of a disaster may well be compatible with the maintenance of normal life for the privileged and thereby understood as failing disaster's subjective criteria. The developments of the past several years, as well as the arguments in this volume, underscore the contested nature of disasters and the frequency with which emergency conditions escape official recognition (see Valentine, Chapter 7 and Miller, Chapter 9).

This uneven recognition reflects public priorities for resource distribution, as official declarations of emergency issue urgent moral demands that open administrative doors enabling state, federal, and international intervention. The recognition that ordinary processes are no longer sufficient for the management of the crisis means that extraordinary funds can be accessed, regular policies bypassed, and more extensive executive actions taken. These opportunities turn the official label of a "public health emergency" into a powerful tool. Consider, for instance, former Massachusetts Governor Deval Patrick's 2014 declaration of the opioid crisis as a state-level public health emergency. The first such declaration concerning opioid addiction, it ushered in some of the broadest policies seen on the issue to date, including prescription monitoring and the banning of a particular painkiller (Wetter et al. 2018). While controversial at the time, Patrick's order prefigured similar actions to publicize and address widespread opioid addiction in other states and, in 2017, at the federal level.[4] The example of the opioid crisis underscores the real potential of an emergency declaration to incite administrative action and galvanize popular support. Under Section 319 of the Public Health Services Act, the Secretary of the U.S. Department of Health and Human Services has renewed COVID-19's status as a national public health emergency every 90 days from January 2020 until May of 2023. At that point, waning support for state intervention into lingering pandemic conditions in the winter and spring of 2023 led to the U.S. Government's decision to end the official public health emergency.

When official emergency status is reached, the actions taken in its name will similarly reflect the priorities of those with administrative power. Certain commonly practiced emergency measures will disproportionately harm disabled people absent adequate proactive intervention. As has been emphasized by disabled activists in the wake of recent natural disasters like hurricanes and wildfires, responses as ostensibly simple as evacuation orders overlook the underlying resources needed to quickly leave one's place of residence, resources that many disabled people, and especially many poor disabled people, lack (Alexander 2015; Weibgen 2014; Nishida 2022). This volume therefore seeks to expose similar complications in the context of epidemic and pandemic disease: crisis standards of care, resource allocation policies, and triage practices number among the many aspects of pandemic planning that, absent specific consideration of the varied needs of disabled communities, will incur deadly consequences for disabled people. Disability advocates across activist, academic, medical, and public policy circles moved quickly in the early phases of the pandemic to articulate these dangers, leading to some significant changes in initial policies.[5] The first triage guidelines to come out of the Alabama Department of Public Health in March 2020, for instance, explicitly excluded certain people with intellectual and developmental disabilities from receiving ventilators should demand for those machines outstrip supply (ALDOPH). Groups including the Alabama Disabilities Advocacy Program and The Arc of the United States filed complaints against these initial guidelines, which were then revised in early April 2020 (see also Ne'eman et al. 2021). *Disability Justice in Public Health Emergencies* builds on the existing efforts of disabled people and disability advocates to articulate emergency planning priorities and response measures that (i) take into account the large body of qualitative and quantitative research on disabled people's health, needs, and experiences, (ii) recognize disabled life as valuable, and (iii) both acknowledge disabled communities as bearers of significant insights and also act upon said insights.

The resources identified in this volume are applicable well beyond officially recognized public health emergencies, whose very determination we and our contributors call into question. As several chapters will note, the conditions of resource scarcity, financial and occupational instability, social precarity, and increased mortality that partially characterize the calamitous harm of public health emergencies have preceded the pandemic for many disabled people (see Savin, Chapter 6 and Valentine, Chapter 7). The levels of poverty experienced by disabled people—more than twice as common than among non-disabled peers, both in the United States and globally—give some indication of this proximity to the crisis explored in the chapters to come (UN Disability and Development; National Council on Disability).[6] Though lacking the recognition, additional funds, and swift administrative actions attending official public health emergencies, many disabled communities have been living under emergency conditions for some time; indeed, the widespread precarity of disabled people is exacerbated by this lack of public support. Emergency conditions will persist for disabled people beyond the official "end" of the pandemic emergency, even as remaining public COVID-19 related funds dry up alongside political and social will for protecting the vulnerable. For a national pandemic response that has already been criticized as leaving responsibilities for risk management to individuals, these diminishing public funds will usher in new levels of privatization.

That the ongoing pandemic puts disabled people, already more likely to live on the edge of emergency due to ableist institutional and social practices, at additional risk for harm demands special consideration. When considered within pandemic planning, an emphasis on the vulnerabilities of disabled people tends to overshadow the active and constructive role that disabled communities play in constructing a more *just future for all*. The next section therefore turns to the framework of disability justice as not only a moral and political imperative, but as a set of strategies and priorities for emergency management.

Disability Justice

Historically, bioethics as a field has had a contentious relationship with critical disability scholarship; we acknowledge this and intend the volume as a critical intervention promoting the work of disability justice within a field that, still today, is too often hostile to it. As the work of disability bioethicists as well as disability theorists working outside of bioethics has frequently underscored, bioethics is held back by its continued privileging of—if not wholesale reliance on—biomedical understandings of disability (Scully 2008, Tremain 2008,

Reynolds and Wieseler 2022). Despite decades of critique, the assumption that disability is nothing more than a problem with an individual body or mind requiring the expertise and intervention of medical providers remains widespread in ways that the essays in this volume detail and criticize. Even where disability issues are nominally included within mainstream bioethics and public health ethics, a focus on systemic ableism, a bold vision of justice, and the voices of disabled communities and activists are too often lacking. This collection therefore contributes to ongoing efforts to strengthen and complicate understandings of disability within healthcare ethics, as well as the practical project of addressing the harms experienced by disabled people during public health crises.

Although the essays in this volume will offer their own framings of disability justice, we here review several different lineages of the concept along with their central commitments. Motivated in part by the persistent failures of the disability rights movement to address the concerns of disabled people of color as well as queer disabled people in the United States, the art-activist collective Sins Invalid developed *disability justice* as an alternative political and theoretical framework (Berne et al. 2018). Without dismissing their legislative gains, which include the protection of disabled people from certain forms of discrimination through Section 504 of the 1973 Rehabilitation Act, the 1975 Individuals with Disabilities Education Act, and the 1990 Americans with Disabilities Act, the disability justice movement highlights the inadequacies of a legislative and specifically anti-discrimination approach to bringing about justice for disabled people.[7] As a political movement grounded in expanding the liberal policies of the U.S. government, the disability rights movement seeks inclusion into the existing body politic without fundamentally altering the terms around which it coheres (see Lajoie 2022). Such a framework seeks to extend political rights—to healthcare, education, employment, and access to public space—but fails to address barriers to equal citizenship that persist even in the face of nominal inclusion or, even more minimally, non-exclusion.

The shortcomings of a disability rights framework become apparent when considering the needs of disabled people who lie outside its purview. For instance, within the education sector, funding for special education programs, as with funding for public education more generally, varies widely depending on the property values of the district to which one is tied (see Conlin & Jalilevand 2015). These economic disparities are demonstrably racialized, resulting in substantial under-resourcing of educational programs for Black and Latinx disabled youth (Marisco 2022). Moreover, the obstacles to access most easily addressed by the ADA represent only a small fraction of the barriers confronted by people with disabilities. In some cases, ramps can be built and sign language interpretation provided, to take just two examples, with minimal alteration of existing public services. The "reasonable accommodation" clause of the ADA, however, denies the necessity of more thoroughgoing transformations that would be required for people with intellectual and developmental disabilities to meaningfully participate in public life (Lajoie 2022; Carlson 2009). Indeed, advocating for inclusion within institutions that have proven so resistant to the concerns of disabled constituents is itself at times a source of objection.

Disability justice theorizing from performance groups like Sins Invalid to, more recently, activist-scholars such as Alice Wong (2020, 2022) and Leah Lakshmi Piepzna-Samarasinha (2018, 2022) has significantly pushed forward conversations concerning how to make the world more just and accessible for all, whether under emergency conditions or not. The guiding principles of this strand of disability justice theorizing reflect a central commitment to solidarity across marginalized identities, disabilities, and movements lacking in the mainstream disability rights movement (Berne et al. 2018). Dating back to the Combahee River Collective, the adoption of an intersectional analysis understands forms of oppression as altering, rather than merely adding to, one another. An intersectional analysis of racism and ableism thus demands a comprehensive, contextual examination of the ways that racism transforms the expression of ableism, as is evident, for example, when racist assumptions about proclivities for violence and disruptiveness impact the identification of behavioral disorders among Black children (Farkas & Morgan 2018). Even further, the intersectionality of disability justice requires seeing disability as extending beyond the cases prioritized by disability rights. An understanding of racialized disablement, as Desiree Valentine's chapter in this volume argues, is key to addressing the production of disability through systemic racism (see Bell 2012; Reynolds 2022; Schalk 2022). Take, for instance, the predominantly Black region of Louisiana where 25% of the country's petrochemicals are produced, nicknamed "Cancer Alley" after the scores of cases that arose among residents who had been exposed to hazardous substances. Recourse through the ADA has yet to be successful in halting the construction of future plants, indicating that a traditional disability rights framework is insufficient to address issues of racialized disablement (Wilson 2022; see also Jampel 2018). As Akemi Nishida notes, an intersectional lens is essential to the study of public health emergencies, since "the COVID pandemic is like a storm that intensifies and speeds up historically developed logics of oppression" (2022, 182). See April Dworetz's arguments in Chapter 4 of this volume for a related analysis of how race and racism, along with other social determinants of health, risk being reproduced by triage protocols.

The disability justice movement's commitment to solidarity is further evidenced by its organizing across movements and disabilities. In addition to the centering of multiply marginalized queer, trans, Black, and Indigenous disabled people, disability justice finds the needs of all disabled people implicated in struggles for environmental sustainability, decarceration, demilitarization, and decolonization (see Ben-Moshe 2020, Erevelles 2016, Meekosha 2011, Puar 2017). The centrality of neoliberal policies of austerity to both the creation and denigration of disability demands that disability justice attend to the economic underpinnings of ableism (Lewis 2023). As demonstrated by Ally Peabody Smith's chapter, disability justice further refuses the marginalization of certain disabilities, especially those deemed most "severe" and "profound," and instead recognizes the incalculable value of all disabled people that frustrates mainstream cost-benefit analyses. Guided by an appreciation of the interdependence between disabled and non-disabled people alike, disability justice strives for collective access and collective liberation for all.

Activist-scholar understandings of disability justice are essential to this volume given both their ambitious visions of social transformation and their concretization in disability-centered emergency management practices on the ground. Leah Lakshmi Piepzna-Samarasinha (2022) and Akemi Nishida (2022) have detailed the efforts of disability justice organizing networks to better protect disabled communities during disasters including, but also preceding, COVID-19. Central to both Piepzna-Samarasinha's and Nishida's arguments are the histories of disabled community care networks made necessary by persistent and systemic failures of public institutions and private organizations to include (let alone prioritize) the needs of disabled people. On top of the costly care and inaccessible clinical environments, deeply rooted assumptions about disability held by providers and integrated into systems protocol make possible institutionalization, loss of parental rights, worsening of medical conditions, and even death real threats (Ben-Moshe 2020). In response to these dangers, and against the isolation experienced by many disabled people as a result of ableism, disabled communities have come together to care for one another's medical, material, and socio-emotional needs. Supporting this longstanding practice and line of scholarship, Sarah Clark Miller's chapter in this volume draws on Piepzna-Samarasinha's concept of *crip doulaship* as a method for supporting COVID long-haulers. But the insights gained from experiences of disability and ableism can also inform emergency management for all: in the midst of disaster and with limited resources, disabled communities "taught all of North America how to make air purifiers out of box fans and a twenty-dollar furnace filter from Lowe's and how to use masks for smoke and then viruses and what the different kinds were" (Piepzna-Samarasinha 2022, 19). Such practical insights demonstrate the kind of creative and accessible interventions borne of disabled experience and activism that are ultimately beneficial to society at large.

Further strands of theorizing justice in ways that center disabled people and communities can be found in feminist theory, philosophy of disability, and critical disability studies. The pioneering scholarship of other authors taken up in this volume, including Eva Feder Kittay, Nirmala Erevelles, Marta Russell, and Jackie Leach Scully, has consistently challenged liberal models of justice. They have been vocal in questioning whether the kinds of social transformation needed to dismantle systemic ableism and promote the multi-faceted flourishing of disabled people can occur within existing institutions. This volume contends that the works of Kittay, Erevelles, Russell, and Scully, among others, contain key resources for thinking critically about what justice demands. These thinkers are not members of the contemporary disability justice movement that grew out of Bay Area organizing, their theories should not be assumed to agree on all points. Indeed, the authors just cited disagree with one another on important points of political strategy and theoretical emphasis. Nonetheless, we consider these disagreements productive for furthering the conversations on what disability justice looks like and how we can get closer to it.

Disability Justice in Public Health Emergencies seeks to put the insights of all of these thinkers in conversation. We understand each of the chapters in this volume to further the project of disability justice in its wider historical emergence, including through sober examination of the tensions between different ways of conceiving it and pursuing it. This volume deploys the concept of 'disability justice' in its most capacious theoretical sense and, at the same time, in the specific practical sense of building a world that is more just for disabled people and, thereby, more just for all people.

The volume's predominant here-and-now actionable focus is on intervening in the emergency procedures of institutional medicine and public health, which, admittedly, departs significantly from the community basis of much DJ organizing. As Guidry-Grimes and Savin note in Chapter 1, the kinds of interventions necessary in the immediate response to a public health emergency often cannot themselves advance the kind of transformative institutional change demanded by projects of disability justice. The essays in this volume go further than established disability rights critiques to advance the issues centered by disability justice. For example, Lajoie's arguments in Chapter 13 show clearly that medical and public health institutions have proven themselves to be untrustworthy to many disabled and otherwise marginalized people. This volume insists that healthcare institutions can *and must* do better. Working through the tensions between disability justice theorizing, bioethics, and institutional healthcare is a necessary component of such a project.

Overview of Contributions

The essays in this volume enumerate, analyze, and offer tools for addressing collective emergencies through the framework of disability justice. Language use, definitions, and political frameworks surrounding disability are all hotly contested. Given the lack of consensus, both locally and globally, over identity-first terms ("I'm a disabled person") and person-first terms ("I'm a person with a disability"), we have not directed contributors to adhere to a particular formulation, and we ourselves purposely alternate between them. Similarly, we have left the authors to articulate definitions of disability and disability justice that best aligns with their work, for we recognize that the demands of context may make a particular definition, model, or framing more suitable than another. We all, however, share the position that neither biomedicine, nor public health hold a monopoly on the definition of disability; individual, social, political, and historical context contributes as much, if not more, to any plausible definition of disability.

Part I, *"Crisis in the Clinic,"* tackles triage processes and crisis standards of care, which emerged as key points of needed intervention for disabled people in the early days of the pandemic. Despite their shared focus on these clinical and administrative practices, the authors in this section each treat different areas of emphasis, collectively composing a fuller and more nuanced approach to accounting for disability in crisis procedures. Katie Savin and Laura Guidry-Grimes present disability justice and disability rights as distinct frameworks with varying recommendations for addressing ableism as reflected in existing triage protocols for public health emergencies. Although a rights-based approach has considerable relevance for revising formal protocols, these actions will not themselves achieve the goal of disability justice. Disability justice—as a radical and intersectional approach demanding a transformation of the background conditions of injustice shaping institutional policies—requires more thoroughgoing change.

Joseph Stramondo critiques Crisis Standards of Care (CSC) protocols, arguing against using quality of life judgments and intensity/duration of treatment metrics and pushing instead for a world in which bioethicists prioritize changing the upstream conditions that shape the downstream effects of systemic injustices. In a similar spirit, April Dworetz argues that a lack of attention to social determinants of health has led to the creation of CSC that perpetuate discrimination on the basis of race and disability specifically. Revised policies influenced by the work of advocates during the early stages of the COVID-19 pandemic have begun to diminish this bias by rejecting categorical exclusions of certain kinds of patients from eligibility, omitting or modifying SOFA scores, and avoiding third-party judgments of an individual's quality of life, among other measures. Continued progress on the revision of CSC, Dworetz contends, will require ongoing input from disability advocates and researchers, substantive involvement of multiply marginalized disabled communities in decision-making, and critical engagement with the most recent population- and individual-level research on disability.

Part II, *"Multiply Marginalized"* highlights specific aspects of systemic ableism and disabled experience that have resulted in increased harm under crisis conditions. Drawing on in-depth interviews with disabled adults in California's San Francisco Bay Area, Katie Savin develops a model of disability as constrained by the workings of the Social Security Administration. Restrictions on the savings and workforce participation of individuals receiving Social Security Disability Income actively place and keep many disabled people in poverty, which further influences the development of individuals' sense of self and strategies for survival. Savin shows the multiple ways in which the COVID-19 pandemic—and even administrative responses intended to relieve some of its negative effects on the most vulnerable members of society—functioned to worsen the living conditions of many disabled people. At the same time, certain pandemic relief programs did result in important gains: Savin argues that efforts like CalFresh's increased benefit generosity can serve as models for extending welfare programs beyond the duration of the current pandemic.

Further interrogating the emergency conditions that preceded the pandemic for multiply marginalized communities, Desirée Valentine takes up the chronic injustices that undergird the racialized production of disability, or, as she puts it, *racialized disablement*. Valentine shows that a declaration of emergency depends on an assumed backdrop of normality where resources are not scarce, institutions function adequately to meet the needs of their constituents, and vulnerability to harm and suffering is not expected. These conditions are simply not met for many people. A simple distinction between normal life and emergency conditions, therefore, elides the ongoing racialized disablement enforced through state policy. Valentine argues that attending to the conjuncture of disability and racism is necessary to the response of emergency conditions both during and beyond the COVID pandemic. Savin and Valentine, respectively, attend to the economic and racialized discrimination that form part and parcel of the ableism experienced by multiply marginalized disabled people. Attending to these co-constitutive axes of oppression is central to the focus of disability justice and essential for effective interventions in crisis management, as well as crisis prevention.

Both the experience and recognition of disability, Nicholas Evans argues, are complicated by the condition of long COVID. On the one hand, given the life-altering changes to physical and cognitive functioning introduced by the syndrome and the forms of exclusion from public life that have followed, there are substantial reasons supporting an understanding of long COVID as a disability. On the other, individual reluctance to embrace a disabled identity, combined with the often invisible and sometimes transient nature of the condition, distance long COVID from some popular understandings of disability. Although long COVID research has received significant investments in a short period of time, scientific, governmental, and popular attention to the condition is likely to remain dependent on the fluctuating recognition of COVID itself as an ongoing threat. Evans argues that reconciling these tensions will require, above all, recognizing the harms of viral pandemics as extending beyond the point of initial infection.

Among the potential harms incurred from rendering disabled people as an afterthought in emergency planning is the shattering of communication strategies necessary for people with profound intellectual disabilities (PID). Though often assumed to be incapable of communication and marginalized even within disability advocacy communities, Ally Peabody Smith shows that non-speaking people may well be able to contribute to the direction of their own care. Smith argues that, because the participation of people with PID in the care process depends on the presence of speaking others with whom they have developed successful, non-verbal modes of communication, reasons of justice demand that emergency protocols make room for the inclusion of these care partners in clinical settings. Disorders of consciousness and intellectual disabilities continue to be marginalized in both bioethics and disability studies, in part because they require greater nuance from those utilizing a social model of disability as their basic framework (see Carlson 2016). Both Chapters 4 and 8 deal with categories of disability and specific diagnoses in ways that may attract criticism over the medicalization of disability. But taking a hybrid approach to understanding disability requires that we acknowl-edge the relevance of biomedicine and the possible utility of clinical categories, even as we refuse to let these dominate the conversation. Both chapters provide essential guidance for providers in cases where negative assumptions about the value of disabled lives are strongest.

Perry Zurn's chapter turns to the recent spread of the "pandemic" as a metaphor for wide-spread and deadly social ills including anti-Black racism, colonialism, and economic inequal-ity. Although the rhetoric has clear appeal and investigation of the confluence of the aforementioned crises is urgently needed, Zurn argues that the over-extended language of "pandemics" hurts more than it helps. Among other effects, such language naturalizes social inequities while setting the collective goal as one of cure, not care. Zurn cautions against both moves insofar as they contribute to damaging discourses of pathologization that critical dis-ability scholarship seeks to remediate. Instead, Zurn finds resources in disability justice's com-mitments to coalition, care, and transformative justice as touchstones for framing emergency response.

Although the entire volume is forward-looking in its articulation of sorely needed actions to improve emergency response, Part III, "*Before the Next Pandemic*," is especially future-oriented. Dealing again with long COVID, Sarah Clark Miller's chapter highlights the need for ongoing societal transformation in the face of this widespread and debilitating post-viral syndrome. As a mass disabling event, Miller argues, the COVID-19 pandemic refuses the neat before-and-after structure of an event and makes a return to "normal" pre-pandemic life both practically impossible and undesirable given the denial of ongoing harm it would require. Picking up where Evans' chapter left off, Miller shows the relevance of Sins Invalid's princi-ples of disability justice for those grappling with long COVID disablement. In particular, she underscores the need for long haulers to learn from and ally with disabled communities rich in the wisdom of confronting systemic ableism.

Emergency response strategies informed by disability justice will need to extend beyond healthcare institutions. In this vein, Kevin Timpe explores what disability justice demands of the American public education system, both during and beyond times of crisis. Because of its necessary link to child development, Timpe boldly—and rightly, we think—argues that edu-cation should be treated as a central domain for bioethical analysis and that bioethicists should be particularly concerned about the disproportionate damage done to disabled stu-dents during the COVID-19 pandemic. Though public education in general was confronted with the massive task of adapting to remote learning, Timpe's research shows that special education programs suffered particularly: where it emerged at all, the provision of virtual special education lagged far behind the establishment of online forms of mainstream educa-tion. Timpe argues that clarified federal guidelines and more district-level accountability are key for minimizing the negative effects of future crises on the educational attainment of dis-abled students.

Finally, Corinne Lajoie considers how a shift toward *institutional trustworthiness* and away from "public trust" better captures the proper locus of responsibility for emergency manage-ment. Lajoie argues that healthcare institutions, in particular, have proven themselves to be untrustworthy through entrenched and ongoing histories of violence that have disproportion-ately damaged disabled people, and especially multiply marginalized disabled people. To begin to remedy the justified losses of trust that have resulted from these harms, Lajoie argues for increased transparency and greater involvement of disabled people in decision-making processes.

Together, the essays in this collection present disability justice as a multifaceted approach that can both diagnose the failures of existing emergency response measures and generate constructive proposals for avoiding such failures in the future. The essays, in other words, articulate how a disability justice approach to emergency preparedness and management provides substantive resources that promise to benefit all. The commitment to intersectionality built into disability justice makes clear that forms of marginalization are multiple and intersecting, resulting in significant variations in what people experience and what kinds of changes are necessary. Disability justice cannot, for instance, focus only on people whose disabilities have been diagnosed and officially recognized; rather, it must consider the logistical and economic barriers to receiving a diagnosis that leave many people without official recognition. Furthermore, attention to marginalized groups is necessary for all emergency planning and management, not merely as a guard against the exacerbation of already existing conditions of scarcity and domination. Those with experience living under emergency conditions already possess vital and transferrable knowledge and skills for navigating them. The recommendations issued here are initial steps toward the substantive involvement of disabled communities and disability advocates in public health emergency planning. If our aim is to achieve a more just emergency response in the future, then we need to heed the insights of disability justice and of disabled people here and now.

Notes

1 Zack herself has written about COVID-19 as a multifaceted series of disasters (2021). See also O'Mathúna, Dranseika, and Gordijn (2018).
2 As reflected in the statistics here, viruses know no national boundaries. Moreover, the dramatically uneven distribution of global wealth and power has meant that emergency conditions and efforts to respond to them have differed widely. This volume takes an admittedly narrow approach by limiting its focus to the U.S. context. Disability justice, however, demands a transnational scope (see Erevelles 2016; Meekosha 2011). We hope to collaborate with colleagues abroad to address the complexities of emergency conditions at a global scale in a sequel to this book.
3 The baseline of inequality that shapes the distribution of emergency burdens from the start motivates ethical approaches like prioritarianism, which seek to address the needs of those worst off first (see Parfit 1995).
4 Compare this response, as many have, with the decidedly carceral and militaristic approach of the War on Drugs in the 1980s and 90s. Notably, the face of the opioid crisis tends to be white while the target of the War on Drugs was almost invariably Black. See also Shachar et al. 2020.
5 See Andrews 2021; Ne'eman et al. 20201; Solomon, Wynia, & Gostin 2020; Guidry-Grimes et al. 2020; and Mello, Persad, and White 2020.
6 In the United States, 36% of disabled people of color live in poverty, compared with 26% of all disabled people (Gupta 2021; National Disability Institute 2020).
7 It is worth mentioning that some disability scholars, including Marta Russell (2002), argue that the passage of the ADA set the disability movement back by accepting its insufficiently transformative focus on anti-discrimination and civil rights law.

Works Cited

Alexander, David. 2015. "Disability and Disaster: An Overview." In *Disability and Disaster: Explorations and Exchanges*, edited by Ilan Kelman and Laura M. Stough, 15–29. Disaster Studies. London: Palgrave Macmillan UK. https://doi.org/10.1057/9781137486004_2
Bell, Christopher M., ed. 2012. *Blackness and Disability: Critical Examinations and Cultural Interventions*. Michigan State University Press.

Ben-Moshe, Liat. 2020. *Decarcerating Disability: Deinstitutionalization and Prison Abolition*. Minneapolis: University of Minnesota Press.

Berne, Patricia, Aurora Levins Morales, David Langstaff, and Sins Invalid. 2018. "Ten Principles of Disability Justice." *WSQ: Women's Studies Quarterly* 46 (1–2): 227–30. https://doi.org/10.1353/wsq.2018.0003

"Biden Team Eyes End of COVID Emergency Declaration and Shift in COVID Team - POLITICO." n.d. Accessed January 11, 2023. https://www.politico.com/news/2023/01/10/biden-covid-public-health-emergency-extension-00077154

Carlson, Licia. 2009. *The Faces of Intellectual Disability: Philosophical Reflections*. Indiana University Press.

Carlson, Licia. 2016. "Feminist Approaches to Cognitive Disability." *Philosophy Compass* 11, no. 10: 541–53. https://doi.org/10.1111/phc3.12350

Conlin, Michael, and Meg Jalilevand. 2015. "Systemic Inequities in Special Education Financing." *Journal of Education Finance*: 83–100.

Curseu, Daniela, Monica Popa, Dana Sirbu, and Ioan Stoian. 2009. "Potential Impact of Climate Change on Pandemic Influenza Risk." *Global Warming*, October, 643–57. https://doi.org/10.1007/978-1-4419-1017-2_45

Davis, Lennard J., ed. 2016. "Is Disability Studies Actually White Disability Studies?" In *The Disability Studies Reader*, 5th ed. Routledge.

Durrheim, David N, Laurence O Gostin, and Keymanthri Moodley. 2020. "When Does a Major Outbreak Become a Public Health Emergency of International Concern?" *The Lancet Infectious Diseases* 20 (8): 887–89. https://doi.org/10.1016/S1473-3099(20)30401-1

Erevelles, Nirmala. 2016. *Disability and Difference in Global Contexts: Enabling a Transformative Body Politic*.

Farkas, George, and Paul L. Morgan. 2018. "Risk and Race in Measuring Special Education Need." *Contexts* 17(4): 72–74. https://doi.org/10.1177/1536504218812876.

Gostin, Lawrence O., Eric A. Friedman, and Sarah A. Wetter. 2020. "Responding to COVID-19: How to Navigate a Public Health Emergency Legally and Ethically." *Hastings Center Report* 50 (2): 8–12. https://doi.org/10.1002/hast.1090

Haffajee, Rebecca, Wendy E. Parmet, and Michelle M. Mello. 2014. "What Is a Public Health 'Emergency'?" *New England Journal of Medicine* 371 (11): 986–88. https://doi.org/10.1056/NEJMp1406167

Jampel, Catherine. 2018. "Intersections of Disability Justice, Racial Justice and Environmental Justice." *Environmental Sociology* 4 (1): 122–35. https://doi.org/10.1080/23251042.2018.1424497

Jennings, Bruce. 2022. "Disaster Response." In *The Routledge Companion to Environmental Ethics*, edited by Benjamin Hale, Andrew Light, Lydia Lawhon. Routledge.

Lajoie, Corinne. 2022. "The Problems of Access: A Crip Rejoinder via the Phenomenology of Spatial Belonging." *Journal of the American Philosophical Association* 8(2): 318–37. https://doi.org/10.1017/apa.2021.6.

Lewis, Talila A. 2023. "Ableism Enables All Forms of Inequity and Hampers All Liberation Efforts." Interview by George Yancy. *Truthout*, January 3, 2023. https://truthout.org/articles/ableism-enables-all-forms-of-inequity-and-hampers-all-liberation-efforts/

Marsico, Richard D. 2021. "The Intersection of Race, Wealth, and Special Education: The Role of Structural Inequities in the IDEA." *NYL Sch. L. Rev.* 66: 207.

Meekosha, Helen. 2011. "Decolonising Disability: Thinking and Acting Globally." *Disability & Society* 26 (6): 667–82. https://doi.org/10.1080/09687599.2011.602860

Ne'eman, Ari, Michael Ashley Stein, Zackary D. Berger, and Doron Dorfman. 2021. "The Treatment of Disability under Crisis Standards of Care: An Empirical and Normative Analysis of Change over Time during COVID-19." *Journal of Health Politics, Policy and Law* 46 (5): 831–60. https://doi.org/10.1215/03616878-9156005

"Newly Released Estimates Show Traffic Fatalities Reached a 16-Year High in 2021 | NHTSA." n.d. Text. Accessed April 6, 2023. https://www.nhtsa.gov/press-releases/early-estimate-2021-traffic-fatalities

Nishida, Akemi. *Just Care: Messy Entanglements of Disability, Dependency, and Desire*. Dis/Color. Philadelphia: Temple University Press, 2022.

O'Mathúna, Dónal P., Vilius Dranseika, and Bert Gordijn, eds. 2018. *Disasters: Core Concepts and Ethical Theories*. Vol. 11. Advancing Global Bioethics. Cham: Springer International Publishing. https://doi.org/10.1007/978-3-319-92722-0

O'Mathúna, Dónal P., Bert Gordijn, and Mike Clarke. 2014. "Disaster Bioethics: An Introduction." In *Disaster Bioethics: Normative Issues When Nothing Is Normal: Normative Issues When Nothing Is Normal*, edited by Dónal P. O'Mathúna, Bert Gordijn, and Mike Clarke, 3–12. Public Health Ethics Analysis. Dordrecht: Springer Netherlands. https://doi.org/10.1007/978-94-007-3864-5_1

Parfit, Derek. 2002. "Equality or Priority?" In *The Ideal of Equality*, edited by Matthew Clayton and Andrew Williams, 81–125. New York.

Piepzna-Samarasinha, Leah Lakshmi. 2022. *The Future Is Disabled: Prophecies, Love Notes, and Mourning Songs*. Vancouver: Arsenal Pulp Press.

Piepzna-Samarasinha, Leah Lakshmi. 2018. *Care Work: Dreaming Disability Justice*. Vancouver: Arsenal Pulp Press.

Puar, Jasbir K. 2017. *The Right to Maim: Debility, Capacity, Disability*. Anima. Durham: Duke University Press.

"Race, Ethnicity and Disability." n.d.

Reynolds, Joel Michael. 2022. "Disability and White Supremacy." *Critical Philosophy of Race* 10 (1): 48–70. https://doi.org/10.5325/critphilrace.10.1.0048

Reynolds, Joel Michael, and Christine Wieseler. "Disability Bioethics: Introduction to The Disability Bioethics Reader." In *The Disability Bioethics Reader*, pp. 1–8. Routledge, 2022.

Russell, Marta. 2002. "What Disability Civil Rights Cannot Do: Employment and Political Economy." *Disability & Society* 17 (2): 117–35. https://doi.org/10.1080/09687590120122288

Schalk, Sami. 2022. *Black Disability Politics*. Duke University Press.

Scully, Jackie Leach. 2008. *Disability Bioethics: Moral Bodies, Moral Difference*. Feminist Constructions. Lanham: Rowman & Littlefield.

Shachar, Carmel, Tess Wise, Gali Katznelson, and Andrea Louise Campbell. 2020. "Criminal Justice or Public Health: A Comparison of the Representation of the Crack Cocaine and Opioid Epidemics in the Media." *Journal of Health Politics, Policy and Law* 45 (2): 211–39. https://doi.org/10.1215/03616878-8004862

Staff, The Petrie-Flom Center. 2021. "Balancing Health Care Rationing and Disability Rights in a Pandemic." *Bill of Health*, January 15, 2021. https://blog.petrieflom.law.harvard.edu/2021/01/15/health-care-rationing-disability-rights-covid/

Stratton, Samuel J. 2020. "COVID-19: Not a Simple Public Health Emergency." *Prehospital and Disaster Medicine* 35 (2): 119–119. https://doi.org/10.1017/S1049023X2000031X

The Lancet Planetary Health. 2021. "A Pandemic Era." *The Lancet. Planetary Health* 5 (1): e1. https://doi.org/10.1016/S2542-5196(20)30305-3

Tremain, Shelley. 2008. "The biopolitics of bioethics and disability." *Journal of Bioethical Inquiry* 5: 101–106.

Weibgen, Adrien A. 2014. "The Right to Be Rescued: Disability Justice in an Age of Disaster." *Yale Law Journal* 124: 2406.

Wetter, Sarah A., James G. Hodge, Danielle Chronister, and Alexandra Hess. 2018 "The Opioid Epidemic and the Future of Public Health Emergencies."

Wilson, Britney. 2022. "Making Me Ill: Environmental Racism and Justice as Disability." SSRN Scholarly Paper. Rochester, NY. https://papers.ssrn.com/abstract=4239837

Wong, Alice, ed. *Disability Visibility: First-Person Stories from the Twenty-First Century*. First Vintage Books edition. New York: Vintage Books, a division of Penguin Random House LLC, 2020.

Wong, Alice. *Year of the Tiger: An Activist's Life*. New York: Vintage Books, a division of Penguin Random House LLC, 2022.

Wu, Zhonglan, David Harrich, Zhongyang Li, Dongsheng Hu, and Dongsheng Li. (2021). "The Unique Features of SARS-CoV-2 Transmission: Comparison with SARS-CoV, MERS-CoV and 2009 H1N1 Pandemic Influenza Virus." *Reviews in Medical Virology* 31(2): e2171. https://doi.org/10.1002/rmv.2171.

Zack, Naomi. *Ethics for Disaster*. Studies in Social, Political, and Legal Philosophy. Lanham (Md.): Rowman & Littlefield, 2009.

Zhu, Zhixing, Xihua Lian, Xiaoshan Su, Weijing Wu, Giuseppe A. Marraro, and Yiming Zeng. 2020. "From SARS and MERS to COVID-19: A Brief Summary and Comparison of Severe Acute Respiratory Infections Caused by Three Highly Pathogenic Human Coronaviruses." *Respiratory Research* 21 (1): 224. https://doi.org/10.1186/s12931-020-01479-w

PART I

Crisis in the Clinic

1

DISABILITY RIGHTS AND DISABILITY JUSTICE AS GESTALT SHIFTS FOR TRIAGE DECISION-MAKING IN A PANDEMIC

Katie Savin and Laura Guidry-Grimes

The COVID-19 pandemic has been a panic-stricken time for disabled people[1] in the United States[2] as a potentially fatal and highly transmissible novel coronavirus created a catastrophe across the globe. People with disabilities feared not just their biological vulnerability to the new virus, but the compounding effects of their marginalized identity. These included concerns that if they were to get sick and need medical help, they could face substandard care, outright denial of care, or even being stripped of their life-sustaining ventilators because of triage protocol proposals favoring younger and healthier patients. From lawsuits to social media posts and Zoom calls to urgent late-night texts, communities of disabled people processed how they heard themselves represented in the media coverage of, and evolving policy around, COVID-19. Disability activist groups signal boosted warnings of rampant ableism, potentially even "new" eugenics,[3] taking place in hospitals, suggesting that they might be denied necessary medical care in the event of overcrowding because their bodies were not valued or prioritized in the pandemic emergency conditions. Hashtags such as #NoICUgenics and #NoBodyIsDisposable were used alongside messaging such as "Don't let #COVID19 triage kill disabled, fat, old, HIV+ and sick people!" (Fat Rose 2020) Text messages circulated to determine if local hospitals were safe to go to, mutual aid networks to share food, medicine, and in-home care were set up, and fears of discrimination deepened across disability communities. Given the legacy of ableism and eugenics in American medicine, these fears were not unfounded. The disproportionate impact on disability communities during COVID-19 marked another era for ableism in public health (*see Shakespeare, Ndagire, and Seketi 2021; Lund and Ayers 2022; Andrews et al. 2021; U.S. National Council on Disability 2021*). How we remember this impact, the nature of the resistance against it, and the progress made toward disability justice as a result have critical implications for the promotion of disability justice in emergency conditions yet to come.

In this chapter, we begin by describing ableism as a systemic and historic form of bias that leads to a cascade of prejudice and disadvantage for disabled people; importantly, ableism runs parallel with other forms of bias such as racism, ageism, and classism. With this necessary background in place, we describe disability rights and disability justice as distinct frameworks for normative analysis and advocacy. We then investigate the central tensions

DOI: 10.4324/9781003502623-3

surrounding the triage of healthcare resources during a pandemic, specifically turning to the evolving moral and political discourse from 2020 to 2022 in relation to COVID-19. We discuss how an emphasis on disability rights was necessary to provide basic protections to persons with disabilities during this public health emergency; however, we also argue that disability *justice* has not been properly elevated or achieved during the pandemic. We then discuss the phenomenon of "informal triage," which leads to denying healthcare resources to disabled persons even when scarcity does not necessitate it. Both formal and informal triage can be especially dangerous for multiply marginalized disabled persons, and a commitment to disability justice is ethically and politically important for reimagining the conditions that lead to formal or informal triage in the first place.

Backdrop of Ableism

Ableism refers to societal attitudes and practices that discriminate against and devalue people who have or are perceived to have disabilities, including physical, intellectual, psychiatric, and other forms of atypicality. The assumption that disabled people need to be fixed and that their lives are inherently and inevitably deficient underlies ableism (*Nario-Redmond 2019; Smith 2023; Asch 2001*). Talila A. Lewis elaborates on the historical, structural, and intersectional aspects in the following definition of 'ableism': "A system that places value on people's bodies and minds based on societally constructed ideas of normalcy, intelligence and excellence. These constructed ideas of normalcy, intelligence and excellence are deeply rooted in anti-Blackness, eugenics and capitalism. This form of systemic oppression leads to people and society determining who is valuable or worthy based on people's appearance and/or their ability to satisfactorily produce, excel and 'behave'" (Lewis 2019). Discrimination, of which ableism is one form, refers to unfair treatment of a person or group of people based on, for example, their perceived or actual disability status. Systemic oppression refers to public policies, institutional and social practices, ideologies, and other norms that work in often reinforcing ways to create and reproduce inequities among groups of people, such as racial groups (Gee and Ford 2011).

Evidence of structural ableism in historic and contemporary medicine and society abounds (Nario-Redmond 2019). A brief glance at events and policies from the past century provides insight into the experiences of people with disabilities being viewed as expendable. Our country has forced sterilizations of people with mental illnesses and developmental disabilities (Buck v. Bell, 274 U.S. 200; Tilley et al. 2012), exploited institutionalized persons with disabilities for research (Rothman and Rothman 1984), and instituted routine use of prenatal genetic testing that raises concerns about devaluing and increasing hostility toward disabled people (McCabe and McCabe 2011; Wasserman and Asch 2005; Saxton 2006) – to name just a few examples. People without disabilities and healthcare professionals tend to rate the quality of disabled persons' lives far lower than disabled people rate their own quality of life (Iezzoni et al. 2021). Feeling that their lives are undervalued, disabled people report fears of inpatient hospital treatment due to concerns of undertreatment, including premature referrals to hospice care and unwanted withdrawal of life-sustaining treatment (Mitchell et al. 2016).

In recent years, public health research in the United States has increasingly recognized that disabled patients experience healthcare disparities compared to their non-disabled counterparts (Krahn, Walker, and Correa-De-Araujo 2015). Thus, people who are disabled had reason for concern that they may be denied critical care during the COVID-19 pandemic. Concerns were magnified for disabled people of color, particularly those who were poor and un- or under-insured, as they face access barriers and health inequities even in non-pandemic circumstances without the same issues of resource scarcity and severely strained healthcare systems (Lund et al. 2020; Gravlee 2020; Maxwell 2020). In part, the ways in which disabled communities and activists perceived and responded to this ableism were reflective of two distinct waves of disability activism and associated scholarship – that of disability rights and disability justice.

Disability Rights and Disability Justice as Distinct Frameworks

Given the pervasiveness of ableism as a background condition for healthcare delivery and other spheres of life, disability communities in the United States have a long history of organized resistance to the discrimination they face. Taking inspiration from the Civil Rights Movement of the 1960s, the disability rights movement (DRM) employed lobbying and protesting tactics in the fight for equal access and basic rights in all areas of public life. The DRM made massive strides in encoding rights for disabled people, such as Section 504 of the Rehabilitation Act; this legislation had been stalled for years and was finally enacted in 1977 after disability activists held sit-ins at federal buildings around the country (Shapiro 2011). When the Americans with Disabilities Act (ADA) of 1990 similarly appeared stuck in the legislature, disability grassroots organizations brought people together for the Capitol Crawl to dramatically demonstrate the lack of access to public buildings. (*Nielsen 2012; Davis 2016; Shapiro 2011*). In the early 2000s, queer and disabled activists of color, who had long felt sidelined from the DRM and the academic field of Disability Studies due to their predominantly white leadership and frequent use of a rights-based framework – with some notable exceptions (e.g., Russell 1998), came together to imagine more radical and intersectional disability activism under the name *disability justice* (DJ). As a "second wave" DRM, the DJ movement perceives ableism as inextricable from other forms of systemic oppression. DJ focuses on how disabilities impact the multiply marginalized members of disability communities, such as those who are incarcerated or undocumented and perhaps lack access to even the rights enshrined in policies such as the ADA, as documented in the seminal DJ primer by Sins Invalid, *Skin, Tooth and Bone: The Basis of Movement is Our People* (2019). Sins Invalid emphasizes that to understand disability justice is to understand "that able-bodied supremacy has been formed in relation to other systems of domination and exploitation. The histories of white supremacy and ableism are inextricably entwined, created in the context of colonial conquest and capitalist domination" (Sins Invalid 2019). The result is a Gestalt shift; the lens of DJ forces a change in our perception of the causes and contours of the oppression of disabled people. Instead of interpreting the whole of the problem in terms of discriminatory practices or dangerous legal silence, DJ prompts us to recognize interlocking oppressive forces on which existing legal systems (and others) rely.

To further clarify the distinctiveness of these movements, take public education as an example. While the DRM made tremendous strides in the education of disabled children through the introduction of Individualized Education Plans with the passage of the Individuals with Disabilities Act (or IDEA, as it was renamed in a 1990 reauthorization, called the Education for All Handicapped Children Act when first enacted in 1975), issues facing many students of color had been neglected. Young Black and Latinx students have increasingly been funneled into the "trapdoor" of special education programs for "behavioral" disabilities that can go on to facilitate school-to-prison pipelines.[4]

As a normative framework and political movement, therefore, we should understand *disability justice* as distinct from *disability rights*. Whereas disability rights focus on the civil rights of people with disabilities within the context of existing economic (capitalist) and legal frameworks, disability justice necessitates dismantling these economic and political systems to remediate disability-based oppression. Because DJ is an intersectional movement at its core, it recognizes that the legal and political systems that can grant civil rights are often not accessible to disabled people at the margins such as those who are people of color, living in poverty, undocumented immigrants, formerly incarcerated, transgender and gender non-conforming, and many others.[5] Thus, while a rights-based movement has been strategic for the DRM, DJ views the legal system as one to overhaul, since its capacity to grant civil rights can also, in turn, incarcerate disproportionate numbers of disabled people of color.

The Gestalt shift toward DJ leads to considering priorities among different communities of disabled persons. In the context of the COVID-19 pandemic, for example, people with disabilities who were incarcerated or undocumented had different concerns and priorities when it came to triaging of care and vaccination access than the general disability population. Community engagement, public health communication, and inclusion strategies can systematically neglect and further marginalize people with disabilities (physical as well as intellectual, developmental, and psychiatric).

Disability justice does not lend itself easily to emergency response, as its fundamental nature is radical: examining the root of the problem of oppression, not the symptoms. It is challenging to apply DJ in a public health emergency because amid the emergency, energy and resources need to go toward survival and crisis management – not reimagining and overhauling existing systems. Applying DJ to pandemic triage protocol, for example, requires questioning the rationale of scarcity and resource distribution, alongside a reimagination and rehauling of everything from a capitalist market economy to a privatized insurance market. During a wildfire, a hurricane, or a pandemic of a novel virus, existing systems need to be optimized to save lives as equitably as possible. Thus, this systemic work needs to be done between emergencies, as we recover from the pandemic.

A focus on disability rights, then, can be justifiable while responding to an actual public health crisis, though we should not be content to stop there. The difficulty in applying disability justice to emergency conditions heightens the importance of collaboration with disability rights and disability justice activism during periods of relative ease, when there is space for healthcare systems and government agencies to explore more systemic routes for change. There is thus a role for both movements and both strategies. But even when considering both disability rights and disability justice in this work, it is important to understand and appreciate their distinctive approaches and visions for diverse people with disabilities.

We turn now to the problem of triage – formal and informal – and how these frameworks for disability advocacy should inform priorities and decision-making.

Avoiding Disability Discrimination in Formal Triage Protocols

Triage, derived from the French word *trier* meaning to sort or separate out, refers to prioritizing patients according to medical urgency and availability of resources. During a public health disaster, a crisis standard of care is triggered after healthcare systems and government agencies determine that conservation, substitution, and adaptation cannot sufficiently expand care capacity for immediate needs, and demand for healthcare resources has outstripped what is

actually available (Berlinger et al. 2020). For the sake of this chapter, this is what we are referring to with the term *formal* triage – triage that is sanctioned, official, based on a codified
process, and necessitated by the scarcity of resources under crisis standards of care. In
responding to COVID-19, the limited, potentially scarce resources that might require triaging
included *space* (intensive care beds), *staff* (critical-care nurses, respiratory therapists, and
other clinicians trained on essential equipment), and *supplies* (personal protective equipment,
ventilators, dialysis machines, pain medications, blood products). Triage protocols must balance several competing considerations: healthcare professionals' duty to care, equitable distribution among a population with diverse health needs, accountability of public agencies and
healthcare systems to serve the public interest, and preserving healthcare systems adequately
so that recovery remains possible after the disaster. No triage system can be "perfect," and
these decisions are tragic, terrible, and haunting for the triage teams and for bedside healthcare professionals. The federal government failed to plan properly for this pandemic or support hospitals and communities in need, and, as a result, hospitals were pushed closer than
necessary to crisis standards of care soon after it spread in the United States (Yong 2020).
COVID-19 was an unparalleled public health disaster.

There are numerous ways to craft a triage protocol according to different value considerations, such as first-come, first-served; lottery; prognosis for short-term survival; prognosis for
long-term survival; life cycles; and values to others in the public health emergency (Daugherty-
Biddison et al. 2017). The challenge in selecting amidst these options is to develop a triage
protocol that will minimize rather than magnify structural discrimination, such as ableism, in
the healthcare system. People with chronic conditions and disabilities face longstanding barriers and inequities in health care (United Nations 2020). As hospitals and public health
authorities devised and shared triage protocols allocating scarce critical-care resources, people with disabilities expressed alarm that these protocols devalue them and exacerbate long-
entrenched ableism in health care. Concerns about ableism in triage protocols include process
and implementation, their design, and their end effects (see Table 1.1).

As can be seen in the quotes in Table 1.1, fear and distrust surrounding triage protocols run
deep, and efforts to minimize ableism have to address each aspect of creating and reviewing
these processes.

Formal complaints alleging disability discrimination in triage protocols were filed in
Washington (The ARC 2020a), Alabama (Alabama Disabilities Advocacy Program 2020),
Tennessee (U.S. Department of Health and Human Services 2020b), Pennsylvania
(U.S. Department of Health and Human Services 2020a), and several other states. The Office
for Civil Rights (OCR) within the U.S. Department of Health and Human Services investi-
gated these complaints and worked with states to revise discriminatory protocols. Disability
activists argued against having categorical exclusions on the basis of disability status, against
incorporating quality of life judgments, against considering long-term life expectancy, and
against reallocating home ventilators (Mello, Persad, and White 2020).[6]

These official complaints and the resulting OCR guidelines are best characterized as a
concern for disability rights, as opposed to disability justice; the actions focused on discrimination on the basis of disability and age but not on other intersecting identities and systems
of disadvantage, such as those related to race, ethnicity, or socio-economic status. Disability
activist organizing efforts leveraged existing civil rights law frameworks that consider social
identity and privilege (or lack thereof) in its component parts, rather than in the intersectional
way disabled lives are lived. Thus, the focus on disability as the target of civil rights violations

TABLE 1.1 Concerns about Ableism Regarding Triage at the Start of the COVID-19 Pandemic

Ableism Concern re: Triage	Example
Process/ implementation *Do the people making these decisions represent disability perspectives?*	"The failure to speak of this vulnerable group is already an indication of how little they seem to matter to people." – Eva Feder Kittay, 2020 "I already knew that for many of the doctors and policymakers that my health depends on, that my transgender, fat, disabled body is simply worth less than others' bodies." – Elliot Kukla, 2020
Design *How could triage criteria put people with disabilities at a disadvantage and perpetuate inequities?*	"They cannot exclude from treatment people whose underlying disabilities mean that they have a lower probability of survival or those who, because of their disabilities, may require a higher level of care." – Disability Rights Education & Defense Fund, 2020 "The mere fact that a person has an intellectual or cognitive disability cannot be a basis for denying care or making that person a lower priority to receive treatment." – Alabama Disabilities Advocacy Program, 2020 "Published descriptions of the goals and flow charts [...] gives priority to treating people who are younger and healthier and leaves those who are older and sicker—people with disabilities—to die." – The Arc, 2020a
Effects *What are long-term implications for people with disabilities?*	"And what happens once we do finally rid the world of this particular mess? Who of the disability community will have met the fate of being remembered as someone sacrificed to save others? And for the disabled people who survive, are we simply supposed to continue on with the knowledge that next time, it might be our turn to be sacrificed?" – Emily Ladau, 2020

neglected how triage protocols can perpetuate inequities for multiply marginalized communities (White and Lo 2021). Disability justice activists argue that people's experiences in healthcare settings will vary such that when compared to a disabled white man, for example, protections for a disabled Black woman will need to address the ways in which ableism in health care rests on white supremacist and patriarchal constructions of normalcy and able-bodiedness. And despite over half a century of civil rights legislation meant to protect disability rights, disabled people continue to experience significant disparities in health and health care, from preventive care to home- and community-based services to acute care (Iezzoni et al. 2022). This distinction between disability rights and disability justice is thus not merely semantic: When researchers, funders, or clinicians erroneously refer to these legal rights-focused actions as demonstrations of disability justice, the term *disability justice* itself loses its distinctive meaning, and it becomes more difficult to use the term properly to emphasize the importance of advocacy from an intersectional standpoint.

To illustrate these different orientations, we can turn to a debate from the early months of the COVID-19 pandemic among mainstream public health ethicists and disability rights advocates regarding the fundamental aim of triage. People in both groups want triage to be equitable, yet they diverged in their conceptions of equity – what it means to be fair and impartial. Several prominent public health ethicists argue that equity requires trying to *maximize the total number of lives saved throughout the course of the pandemic* (Emanuel et al. 2020). For many in the disability community, however, equity means that people with disabilities and chronic illnesses have the *same chance of receiving maximum health care as their nondisabled peers* (Savin and Guidry-Grimes 2020; Guidry-Grimes et al. 2020). In a public health context, medical criteria related to critical care survivability are scientifically pertinent evidence and not considered discriminatory. Many people with disabilities, who have lived experiences of inequitable treatment and lack of access based on their embodied and physiological differences, perceive the same medical criteria as the usual grounds for discrimination.

With different perspectives on equity and therefore different goals of triage, the methods of triage that the two groups advocate for also differ. Many in the disability community favor methods that eliminate consideration of underlying health conditions and do not address short- or long-term survivability (*Stramondo 2020*). A Disability Rights Education & Defense Fund (DREDF) policy brief explicitly makes this argument and advises, "When dealing with patients with a similar level of treatment urgency, providers should maintain their existing practice of 'first come, first served,' rather than prioritizing people who would require the fewest resources" (DREDF 2020). Ari Ne'eman, a disability activist who provided consultation for OCR later in the pandemic, also argued (2020) in *The New York Times* that a first come, first served policy should be followed for all healthcare resources, including ventilators, regardless of any potential scarcity in the pandemic. Others favor a lottery (Shapiro 2020a). Providing care on a 'first come, first serve' basis in the context of activated triage protocol may reduce the risk of discrimination based on age and disability but could exacerbate existing healthcare inequities based on race or ethnicity and socio-economic status. Social determinants of health that have led to worse health outcomes both before and throughout the pandemic for people in racial and ethnic minoritized groups and in lower socio-economic statuses, such as lack of transportation access, distrust in medical systems, lower rates of health literacy, among many others, are common causes of delayed treatment in these communities (Tolchin, Hull, and Kraschel 2021). Thus, advocacy for a 'first come, first serve' triage protocol could not be reasonably deemed disability justice, nor would any advocacy aimed toward ameliorating disability discrimination that did not consider the broader context of social determinants of health impacting lower-income communities and communities of color.

The fight against disability discrimination in formal triage was necessary in the COVID-19 pandemic. Disability activists engaged in this work made important albeit incomplete progress for the protection of disabled people in the event that crisis standards of care were to be enacted. Even if crisis standards were not activated in any given state or healthcare system, the conversation about disability rights in a pandemic spread across academia, the national press, and even in some clinical spaces that routinely neglect the topic of disability rights, such as hospital ethics committees and enterprise policy committees. It is not our intent to downgrade this important anti-discrimination work, which is made even more extraordinary given the crucible of the pandemic, but we also have to be frank about what was and was not achieved here. Triage protocol adjustments to prevent outright discrimination is still a low bar to set – it is necessary but *by no means sufficient* for just treatment of disabled people in a public health crisis. This point is well-recognized by disability communities but not always appreciated by people outside of those communities. To help elucidate this issue, we turn now to the phenomenon of informal triage, which is an area of potentially ableist decision-making that can go unnoticed both before and during a public health crisis.

Informal Triage and Disability Justice

When demand for resources starts to outstrip supply beyond usual operations, healthcare systems can enter *contingency* standards before they reach *crisis* standards.[7] As put by the Institute of Medicine in 2009: "The delivery of care in the setting of contingency surge response seeks to provide patient care that remains *functionally equivalent* to conventional care" (14, emphasis added). This framing can make it appear that dangers to current and would-be patients are avoided prior to crisis standards, but the COVID-19 pandemic demonstrated, repeatedly, the ethical complexities and ableism that can still arise (Alfandre et al. 2021). The idea that care would remain "functionally equivalent" is perhaps one of the most misleading and hazardous suggestions in pandemic planning, for it neglects the foreseeable disproportionate impacts of a pandemic on multiply marginalized communities that already experience inequities in health care. Informal triage raises concerns regardless of whether crisis standards of care are enacted, and it is one way in which care can be far less than "functionally equivalent" for these populations.

Generally, "informal triage" captures a range of practices that can vary in how problematic or justifiable they are in context. For example, this term can be applied anytime non-clinical groups, such as reception staff or designated expert patients, screen people to determine whether they should be seen by clinicians (Rodrigues et al. 2022; Landes et al. 2017). During the COVID-19 pandemic, informal triage also meant that some patients were automatically declined access to critical care resources, meaning they were also denied individualized assessment by anyone in a position of medical gatekeeping. Informal triage is also not necessarily based on full information about surge capacity, the most up-to-date evidence about the public health disaster or treatment options, or sanctioned processes. Consider the following report from France:

> Bedside triage was less prevalent than an upstream, informal triage made by declining to transfer older patients to an ICU (or even sometimes to a hospital) [...] Triage was de facto taking place at the first responder's level. A medical argument sometimes invoked was that older people would not do well on a ventilator (a similar informal policy existed regarding disabled people – particularly those in institutions – who would often not be transferred to hospitals).
>
> *(Orfali 2020, 677–678)*

Even if a disabled person made it to a hospital for assessment, there were concerns and reports during the pandemic that "individual medical providers have made their own decisions about allocating scarce medical treatment apart from any formalized crisis standards of care" (Judge David L. Bazelon Center for Mental Health Law et al. 2021, 3). This last form of informal triage can be particularly pernicious because it may not appear to be a triage-related decision at all – healthcare professionals regularly decide what therapies to offer and how aggressively to continue certain treatments.

When a public health crisis makes healthcare professionals increasingly concerned about exceeding surge capacity and having to work in the nightmare scenario that is crisis standards of care, they may become especially conservative in their use of resources – especially with patients whose quality of life seems low, whose life expectancy seems shorter than "average," or who would use multiple resources that could become scarce. Conserving resources in these instances may seem to be the prudent and ethically justified decision, a way for individual providers to do their part as responsible stewards in a public health disaster. Informal triage could also occur when healthcare professionals misunderstand the process for triage decision-making or the status of the crisis in their clinical space, so they make decisions that do not follow the established procedure or criteria. Ableism, racism, classism, and other forms of implicit bias can pervade this decision-making, however, as seen in the above examples. And because it is informal, this type of triage can fall below the radar for reporting, accountability, and transparency.

It is unclear how many clinical and non-clinical staff felt empowered to make informal triage decisions outside of crisis standards of care being enacted. The lack of data and published accounts of informal triage in the pandemic also mean that future planning for public health emergencies, at national and local levels, could overlook this issue altogether. For disability communities advocating for disability justice, however, the possibility of informal triage during a pandemic – and its normalization beyond the pandemic – remain consistent concerns. In a report published by a collective of disability-affiliated organizations, formal and informal triage during the COVID-19 pandemic were analyzed for their potential for intersectional discrimination and the perpetuation of inequities. They highlight, for example, the well-publicized stories of Michael Hickson and Sarah McSweeney. The Michael Hickson case "is just one example of a tragedy that raises questions about the impact of race and disability bias in decisions about who receives life-sustaining treatment" for reasons that were not dictated by crisis standards of care (Judge David L. Bazelon Center for Mental Health Law et al. 2021). Michael Hickson had multiple disabilities, including quadriplegia and cortical blindness, before he fell ill due to COVID-19. There were several troubling aspects related to his case, and at a critical point, his physician was recorded telling Mrs. Hickson that further treatment would be "futile" due to Michael Hickson's low quality of life with his disabilities. Michael Hickson was ultimately transitioned to comfort care and hospice services over objections of the family, and he died (Shapiro 2020b). Sarah McSweeney also had several disabilities before being admitted to a hospital for high fever and COVID-19. Even though she had a POLST (Physician Orders for Life-Sustaining Treatment, a portable form of advance care planning) that explicitly stated a preference to be full code, her physicians urged she become DNR. They also denied her a ventilator, despite its being the evident standard of care for her condition, and even though her hospital did not have a shortage of ventilators. Following many disagreements with the medical team regarding her goals of care and conversations with incredulous hospital staff about her quality of life, Sarah McSweeney died in the hospital. (Shapiro 2020c).

Issues of informal triage cannot be as readily addressed through a rights-based framework because they are, by nature, not codified, so there is no institutionalized mechanism to ban them. Instead, inappropriate informal triage might be better addressed through a disability justice framework that examines a problem at its roots, using an intersectional lens, and informed by those most impacted by the issue. At the roots of informal triage, we find multiple types of overt discrimination and implicit bias that include ableism, racism, and classism. Responding to informal triage does require grappling with the fact that we are likely unaware of the majority of incidences. Thus, healthcare systems and training programs should raise awareness of the risks of informal triage, personal and institutional biases that may be involved, and some of the key decision-making points when it tends to occur; hopefully this will help healthcare professionals identify and analyze these practices, so they no longer fall beneath the radar. Clinical policies should also try to ensure some level of oversight and accountability for sensitive decisions that may reflect interpersonal or systemic bias, such as with "futility" determinations – which will help patients receive equitable care even in non-pandemic conditions (U.S. National Council on Disability 2019). If states mandate transparency with hospitals' real-time surge capacities for the public, this information could also potentially help patients and their families avoid hospitals that are especially strained and more prone (potentially) to informal triage.

Recommendations

As public health disasters become more chronic due to global warming and conflict, it will be especially important to plan appropriately so as to limit the strains that lead to formal and informal triage as much as possible.[8] This planning should take into consideration the socio-historical context of health inequities and how the burdens of these disasters disproportionately affect disabled people. We offer suggestions to bioethicists and healthcare providers for concrete strategies on using a disability justice lens to collaborate with disability activists and communities during and between emergency conditions.

- Conduct an institutional assessment of informal triage through staff and patient surveys. Identify key decision-making junctures that could permit inappropriate and unsanctioned informal triage. Develop monitoring and tracking systems for informal triage to which patients as well as non-clinical and clinical staff can report. Ensure that disability status, type of disability, and needed accommodations are among the demographic data collected on all patients at all levels of care (Akobirshoev et al. 2022). Provide staff trainings on implicit bias and discrimination in the context of informal triage.
- Hire people from disability communities from a variety of backgrounds to provide disability-related education, including intersectional anti-ableism trainings, in academic settings for health professionals in training as well as in clinical settings for continuing education. Ideally, providers who treat people with disabilities will have experience interacting with the disability community when they are not in the patient context.
- Ask individuals/communities to participate in your organizations in ongoing ways, not just for one-off events (e.g., sitting on boards, ethics committees, etc.). This will help build trust, decrease perceived or actual conflicts of interest, and allow for input on more structural decisions than is allowed for during emergency conditions as well as incorporate the principle of leadership of the most impacted.
- Offer compensation for labor. Many activities that professionals may consider "service" bring them credit in their official capacities, such as speaking engagements and writing or co-authorship opportunities. However, for many disabled people not in academic or health professions, these activities will not bring them the same usable credit. People with disabilities have historically been and continue to be marginalized and exploited in the labor market, and it is critical to avoid reproducing this dynamic in community partnerships. Work with individuals as much as possible to find acceptable options, such as by offering all-purpose gift cards in lieu of checks, for those who may encounter administrative obstacles to receiving employment-based income due to Social Security policies that penalize work activity.

- Use platforms when hospital communities come together, such as Grand Rounds, to discuss patient cases such as the Hickson case. Increase awareness and understanding of ableism and how it may manifest in clinical practice, even among well-intentioned professionals.
- Increase pipelines to healthcare professions and clinical bioethics for people with disabilities through the development of targeted recruitment activities, scholarships, and mentoring programs.
- While in a non-emergency period, revisit triage protocols and other crisis-related institutional policies. In a public and accessible online forum, make proposals for triage processes available for comment from the community (National Association for the Deaf). Reach out to local community groups representing different marginalized groups, for example, disabled, immigrant, queer/trans groups to provide input.
- Regional agreements are needed proactively for resource-sharing systems and load balancing to have a more equitable process for preventing triage decisions in the first place; such a system will help prevent placing a greater burden on low-resource areas, which can exacerbate inequities for racial minorities, people with disabilities, and other disadvantaged patients in those areas (White, Villarroel, and Hick 2021).
- Provide funding toward innovation in critical care resources to expand capacity during contingency and crisis standards of care. Innovations should not directly or indirectly put disabled people at greater risk, for example, re-engineering community ventilators commandeered from care facilities for use in intensive care units (Reynolds, Guidry-Grimes, and Savin 2021).
- Humanizing is an advocacy strategy disability communities used prior to and during the pandemic to lessen their chances of facing disability-based discrimination or informal triage of care. In the context of health care, humanizing could look like decorating one's hospital room with pictures of the patient with disabilities in the context of their everyday life, such as with friends and family, at work, or out in the community. Particularly in the context of patients with communication disabilities or those who are unable to communicate due to their current medical condition, humanizing might also involve posting a brief message to healthcare providers such as, "Hi, my name is Katie. I'm a social work professor and disability activist. I love to garden and spend time with my cat, Stevie. Thank you for your care." This imagery and messaging are intended to counteract the dehumanizing of people with disabilities that can take place in all parts of society, but especially in health settings. The group #NoBodyIsDisposable describes this as a "Connection Kit" in their "guide to surviving COVID-19 triage protocols" (NoBody Is Disposable Coalition 2020). Clinical bioethicists and allied health professionals such as medical social workers can support patients and families with these efforts and even incorporate a brief personal descriptor of patients in their chart notes.

Acknowledgments

Some sections of this chapter appeared in our co-authored blog post, "Confronting Disability Discrimination During the Pandemic," published by the *Hastings Bioethics Forum*. We are grateful to Nancy Berlinger, Joseph Stramondo, Erik Parens, Norine McGrath, and Susan Gilbert for their insights and feedback as we wrote this blog post. This chapter benefited from recommendations from the editors, for which we are grateful.

Notes

1 There is continued debate about identity-first versus person-first language in disability studies and activism; we alternate between the terms in this chapter out of deference to the different perspectives on this issue.
2 We will focus on the U.S. context, though many of our concerns and arguments apply to other countries as well.
3 There are arguments that the United States never stopped its eugenic policies and thinking, so eugenics is not really new in this context. See Ordover 2003.
4 Annamma and colleagues explore this issue using Disability Critical Race Theory (DisCrit) to provide a critical structural analysis of how educational and carceral system policies at the state and federal levels have led to overrepresentation of youth of color in school discipline and special education programs which lead to their subsequent policing and involvement in the juvenile justice systems. See, Annamma, Morrison, and Jackson, 2014; Erevelles, 2014; Annamma, Connor, and Ferri, 2013.
5 For more, see Sins Invalid 2019; Chin 2021.
6 This is not a comprehensive list of the discrimination complaints that were filed. For example, some disability rights groups also argued against any consideration of short-term survival outside of immediate survival potential from COVID-19. OCR also addressed disability discrimination concerns regarding aspects of the pandemic that did not directly relate to triage protocols, such as hospital visitation policies and telehealth services. See Disability Rights Connecticut 2020.
7 The nature of the public health crisis would make a difference for whether a healthcare system transitioned into contingency standards before crisis standards. A sudden natural disaster, such as a hurricane or tornado, is importantly different from a gradually worsening pandemic in this way.
8 The problem of increasing *chronicity* with public health disasters – as well as the importance of macroallaction planning to balance public health and equity – was part of a panel with Chad Priest, Douglas White, and Laura Guidry-Grimes at the 2023 Carfang Nursing Ethics Conference.

Works Cited

Akobirshoev, Ilhom, Michael Vetter, Lisa I. Iezzoni, Sowmya R. Rao, and Monika Mitra. 2022. "Delayed Medical Care and Unmet Care Needs Due to the COVID-19 Pandemic Among Adults with Disabilities in the US." *Health Affairs* 41 (10): 1505–1512. https://doi.org/10.1377/hlthaff.2022.00509

Alabama Disabilities Advocacy Program. 2020. "Complaint of Alabama Disabilities Advocacy Program and The Arc of the United States," March 24, 2020. https://www.centerforpublicrep.org/wp-content/uploads/2020/03/AL-OCR-Complaint_3.24.20.docx.pdf?fbclid=IwAR2EZ8TJTGygD7Lhl5Q_QX5JX0Es3DHrtVbhmn1GaNBS1UZh9bmq2E_D_S8

Alfandre, David, Virginia Ashby Sharpe, Cynthia Geppert, Mary Beth Foglia, Kenneth Berkowitz, Barbara Chanko, and Toby Schonfeld. 2021. "Between Usual and Crisis Phases of a Public Health Emergency: The Mediating Role of Contingency Measures." *The American Journal of Bioethics* 21 (8): 4–16.

Andrews, Erin E., Kara B. Ayers, Kathleen S. Brown, Dana S. Dunn, and Carrie R. Pilarski. 2021. "No Body Is Expendable: Medical Rationing and Disability Justice during the COVID-19 Pandemic." *American Psychologist* 76: 451–61. https://doi.org/10.1037/amp0000709

Annamma, Subini, David Connor, and Beth Ferri. 2013. "Dis/Ability Critical Race Studies (DisCrit): Theorizing at the Intersections of Race and Dis/Ability." *Race Ethnicity and Education* 16 (1): 1–31. https://doi.org/10.1080/13613324.2012.730511

Annamma, Subini, Deb Morrison, and Darrell Jackson. 2014. "Disproportionality Fills in the Gaps: Connections between Achievement, Discipline and Special Education in the School-to-Prison Pipeline." *Berkeley Review of Education* 5 (1): 53–87.

Asch, Adrienne. 2001. "Disability, Bioethics, and Human Rights." In *Handbook of Disability Studies*, edited by Gary L. Albrecht, Katherine D. Seelman, Michael Bury, 297–326. Thousand Oaks, CA: Sage Publications.

Berlinger, Nancy, Matthew Wynia, Tia Powell, D. Micah Hester, Aimee Milliken, Rachel Fabi, Felicia Cohn, Laura K. Guidry-Grimes, Jamie Carlin Watson Lori Bruce, Elizabeth J. Chuang, Grace Oei, Jean Abbott, Nancy Piper Jenks. 2020. "Ethical Frameworks for Health Care Institutions & Guidelines for Institutional Ethics Services Responding to the Coronavirus Pandemic: Managing

Uncertainty, Safeguarding Communities, Guiding Practice." *The Hastings Center*, March 16, 2020. https://www.thehastingscenter.org/ethicalframeworkcovid19

Buck v. Bell, 274 U.S. 200 (1927).

Chin, Natalie M. 2021. "Centering Disability Justice." *Syracuse Law Review* 71: 683–749.

Davis, Lennard J. 2016. *Enabling Acts: The Hidden Story of How the Americans with Disabilities Act Gave the Largest US Minority Its Rights.* Beacon Press.

Daugherty-Biddison, Lee, Howard Gwon, Alan Regenberg, Monica Schoch-Spana, Eric Toner. 2017. "Maryland Framework for the Allocation of Scarce Life-sustaining Medical Resources in a Catastrophic Public Health Emergency." *Bioethicstoday*, 24 August 2017. https://bioethicstoday.org/wp-content/uploads/2020/03/Daugherty-Maryland-framework-PH-emergency-2017.pdf?x41592

Disability Rights Education & Defense Fund (DREDF). 2020. "Preventing Discrimination in the Treatment of COVID-19 Patients: The Illegality of Medical Rationing on the Basis of Disability." *DREDF*, March 25, 2020. https://dredf.org/the-illegality-of-medical-rationing-on-the-basis-of-disability/

Disability Rights Connecticut. 2020. "Illegal Disability Discrimination Concerning Hospital COVID-19 Visitation Policies." *DRC*, May 4, 2020. https://www.ndrn.org/wp-content/uploads/2020/05/CT-OCR-visitor-policy-cmplt-FINAL-5.4.20-.pdf

Emanuel, Ezekiel J., Govind Persad, Ross Upshur, Beatriz Thome, Michael Parker, Aaron Glickman, Cathy Zhang, Connor Boyle, Maxwell Smith, and James P Phillips. 2020. "Fair Allocation of Scarce Medical Resources in the Time of COVID-19." *New England Journal of Medicine* 382 (21): 2049–2055.

Erevelles, Nirmala. 2014. "Crippin' Jim Crow: Disability, Dis-Location, and the School-to-Prison Pipeline." In *Disability Incarcerated: Imprisonment and Disability in the United States and Canada*, edited by Liat Ben-Moshe, Chris Chapman, and Allison C. Carey, 81–99. New York: Palgrave Macmillan US. http://doi.org/10.1057/9781137388476_5

Fat Rose, (@FatRoseAction). 2020. "Don't Let #COVID19 Triage Kill Disabled, Fat, Old, HIV+ and Sick People! FIGHT FOR OUR LIVES." Twitter, May 29, 2020, 3:09pm. https://twitter.com/FatRoseAction/status/1244386194563063808

Gee, Gilbert C., and Chandra L. Ford. 2011. "Structural Racism and Health Inequities: Old Issues, New Directions1." *Du Bois Review: Social Science Research on Race* 8 (1): 115–132.

Gravlee, Clarence C. 2020. "Systemic Racism, Chronic Health Inequities, and COVID-19: A Syndemic in the Making?" *American Journal of Human Biology* 32 (5): e23482. https://doi.org/10.1002/ajhb.23482

Guidry-Grimes, Laura, Katie Savin, Joseph A. Stramondo, Joel Michael Reynolds, Marina Tsaplina, Teresa Blankmeyer Burke, Angela Ballantyne, Eva Feder Kittay, Devan Stahl, Jackie Leach Scully, Rosemarie Garland-Thomson, Anita Tarzian, Doron Dorfman, Joseph J. Fins. 2020. "Disability Rights as a Necessary Framework for Crisis Standards of Care and the Future of Health Care." *Hastings Center Report* 50 (3): 28–32. https://doi.org/10.1002/hast.1128

Iezzoni, Lisa I., Michael M. McKee, Michelle A. Meade, Megan A. Morris, and Elizabeth Pendo. 2022. "Have Almost Fifty Years of Disability Civil Rights Laws Achieved Equitable Care?" *Health Affairs* 41 (10): 1371–1378. https://doi.org/10.1377/hlthaff.2022.00413

Iezzoni, Lisa I., Sowmya R. Rao, Julie Ressalam, Dragana Bolcic-Jankovic, Nicole D. Agaronnik, Karen Donelan, Tara Lagu, and Eric G. Campbell. 2021. "Physicians' Perceptions of People with Disability and Their Health Care." *Health Affairs* 40 (2): 297–306. https://doi.org/10.1377/hlthaff.2020.01452

Institute of Medicine. 2009. *Guidance for establishing crisis standards of care for use in disaster situations: A letter report.* Washington, DC: The National Academies Press.

Invalid, Sins. 2019. *Skin, Tooth, and Bone–the Basis of Movement Is Our People: A Disability Justice Primer*, 2nd ed. Berkeley, CA: Sins Invalid.

Judge David L. Bazelon Center for Mental Health Law, Lawyer's Committee for Civil Rights Under Law, Disability Rights Education & Defense Fund (DREDF), The Arc, Center for Public Representation, Autistic Self Advocacy Network, Justice in Aging, et al. 2021. "Examining How Crisis Standards of Care May Lead to Intersectional Medical Discrimination Against COVID-19 Patients." June 23, 2021. https://thearc.org/resource/intersectional-guide-to-crisis-care

Kittay, Eva Feder. 2020. "Invisible Vulnerables." *Official Blog of IJFAB: The International Journal of Feminist Approaches to Bioethics*, March 29, 2020. https://www.ijfab.org/blog/2020/03/invisible-vulnerables/?fbclid=IwAR0hPXBmBAq7krRbExD-fDgd4EA_V44axqtj1Xm7_r-OtJ25da5Fw_LH3gE

Krahn, Gloria L., Deborah Klein Walker, and Rosaly Correa-De-Araujo. 2015. "Persons with Disabilities as an Unrecognized Health Disparity Population." *American Journal of Public Health* 105 (S2): S198–206. https://doi.org/10.2105/AJPH.2014.302182

Kukla, Elliot. 2020. "My Life Is More 'Disposable' During This Pandemic." *New York Times*, March 19, 2020. https://www.nytimes.com/2020/03/19/opinion/coronavirus-disabled-health-care.html

Ladau, Emily. 2020. "As A Disabled Person, I'm Afraid I May Not Be Deemed Worth Saving from The Coronavirus." *HuffPost*, March 25, 2020. https://www.huffpost.com/entry/coronavirus-healthcare-rationing-medical-ethics-disability_n_5e7a2b0dc5b6f5b7c54bb117?ncid=engmodushpmg 00000003&fbclid=IwAR1o2nriHYv5gC-Saa4ARa3HOhsFs9GrVHUiGME_hWvlMcm EPXfT2i--SIM

Landes, Megan, Courtney Thompson, Edson Mwinjiwa, Edith Thaulo, Chrissie Gondwe, Harriet Akello, and Adrienne K. Chan. 2017. "Task Shifting of Triage to Peer Expert Informal Care Providers at a Tertiary Referral HIV Clinic in Malawi: A Cross-Sectional Operational Evaluation." *BMC Health Services Research* 17 (1): 1–7.

Lewis, Talia A. 2019. "Longmore Lecture: Context, Clarity & Grounding." *Talia A. Lewis Blog*, March 5, 2019. https://www.talilalewis.com/blog/longmore-lecture-context-clarity-grounding

Lund, Emily M., and Kara B. Ayers. 2022. "Ever-Changing but Always Constant: 'Waves' of Disability Discrimination during the COVID-19 Pandemic in the United States." *Disability and Health Journal* 15 (4): 101374. https://doi.org/10.1016/j.dhjo.2022.101374

Lund, Emily M., Anjali J. Forber-Pratt, Catherine Wilson, and Linda R. Mona. 2020. "The COVID-19 Pandemic, Stress, and Trauma in the Disability Community: A Call to Action." *Rehabilitation Psychology* 65 (4): 313. http://doi.org/10.1037/rep0000368313

Maxwell, Connor. 2020. "Coronavirus Compounds Inequality and Endangers Communities of Color." *Center for American Progress*, March 7, 2020. https://www.americanprogress.org/article/coronavirus-compounds-inequality-endangers-communities-color/

McCabe, Linda L., and Edward R. B. McCabe. 2011. "Down Syndrome: Coercion and Eugenics." *Genetics in Medicine* 13: 708–710. https://doi.org/10.1097/GIM.0b013e318216db64

Mello, Michelle M, Govind Persad, and Douglas B White. 2020. "Respecting Disability Rights—toward Improved Crisis Standards of Care." *New England Journal of Medicine* 383 (5): e26.

Mitchell, Suzanne E., Gabriela M. Weigel, Sabrina K.A. Stewart, Morgan Mako, and John F. Loughnane. 2016. "Experiences and Perspectives on Advance Care Planning among Individuals Living with Serious Physical Disabilities." *Journal of Palliative Medicine* 20 (2): 127–133. https://doi.org/10.1089/jpm.2016.0168

Nario-Redmond, Michelle R. 2019. *Ableism: The Causes and Consequences of Disability Prejudice*. John Wiley & Sons.

National Association for the Deaf. n.d. "COVID-19: Deaf and Hard of Hearing Communication Access Recommendations for the Hospital." *NAD*. https://www.nad.org/covid19-communication-access-recs-for-hospital/

Ne'eman, Ari. 2020. "'I Will Not Apologize for My Needs.'" *New York Times*, March 23, 2020. https://www.nytimes.com/2020/03/23/opinion/coronavirus-ventilators-triage-disability.html

Nielsen, Kim E. 2012. *A Disability History of the United States*. Beacon Press.

NoBody Is Disposable Coalition. 2020. "Know Your Rights Guide to Surviving COVID-19 Triage Protocols." *#NoBodyIsDisposable*, July 28, 2020. https://nobodyisdisposable.org/know-your-rights/

Office of Civil Rights. 2020. "Civil Rights and COVID-19." U.S. Health and Human Services, April 29, 2020. https://www.hhs.gov/civil-rights/for-providers/civil-rights-covid19/index.html

Ordover, Nancy. 2003. *American Eugenics: Race, Queer Anatomy, and the Science of Nationalism*. Minneapolis, MN: University of Minnesota Press.

Orfali, Kristina. 2020. "What Triage Issues Reveal: Ethics in the COVID-19 Pandemic in Italy and France." *Journal of Bioethical Inquiry* 17 (4): 675–679.

Reynolds, Joel Michael, Laura Guidry-Grimes, and Katie Savin. 2021. "Against Personal Ventilator Reallocation." *Cambridge Quarterly of Healthcare Ethics* 30 (2): 272–284. https://doi.org/10.1017/S0963180120000833.

Rodrigues, Daniela, Noemi Kreif, Kavitha Saravanakumar, Brendan Delaney, Mauricio Barahona, and Erik Mayer. 2022. "Formalising Triage in General Practice towards a More Equitable, Safe, and Efficient Allocation of Resources." *BMJ* 377: e070757. https://doi.org/10.1136/bmj-2022-070757

Rothman, David J., and Sheila M. Rothman. 1984. *The Willowbrook Wars: Bringing the Mentally Disabled into the Community*. New York City: Harper & Row Publishers.

Russell, Marta. 1998. *Beyond Ramps: Disability at the End of the Social Contract: A Warning from an Uppity Crip*. Common Courage Press.

Savin, Katie, and Laura Guidry-Grimes. 2020. "Confronting Disability Discrimination During the Pandemic." *Hastings Bioethics Forum*, April 2, 2020.

Saxton, Marsha. 2006. "Disability Rights and Selective Abortion." In *The Disability Studies Reader*, 2nd ed. edited by Lennard Davis, 105–116. London: Routledge Press.

Shakespeare, Tom, Florence Ndagire, and Queen E Seketi. 2021. "Triple Jeopardy: Disabled People and the COVID-19 Pandemic." *The Lancet* 397, no. 10282: 1331–1333.

Shapiro, Joseph. 2011. *No Pity: People with Disabilities Forging a New Civil Rights Movement*. New York, NY: Three Rivers Press.

Shapiro, Joseph. 2020a. "Disability Groups File Federal Complaint About COVID-19 Care Rationing Plans." *National Public Radio*, March 23, 2020. https://www.npr.org/2020/03/23/820303309/disability-groups-file-federal-complaint-about-covid-19-care-rationing-plans

Shapiro, Joseph. 2020b. "One Man's COVID-19 Death Raises the Worst Fears of Many People with Disabilities." *National Public Radio*, July 31, 2020. https://www.npr.org/2020/07/31/896882268/one-mans-covid-19-death-raises-the-worst-fears-of-many-people-with-disabilities

Shapiro, Joseph. 2020c. "As Hospitals Fear Being Overwhelmed By COVID-19, Do the Disabled Get the Same Access?" *National Public Radio*, December 14, 2020. https://www.npr.org/2020/12/14/945056176/as-hospitals-fear-being-overwhelmed-by-covid-19-do-the-disabled-get-the-same-acc

Shapiro, Joseph 2020d. "Oregon Hospitals Told Not to Withhold Care Because Of a Person's Disability." *National Public Radio*, December 21, 2020. https://www.npr.org/2020/12/21/948697808/oregon-hospitals-told-not-to-withhold-care-because-of-a-persons-disability

Smith, Leah. 2023. "#Ableism." *Center for Disability Rights*. cdrnys.org/blog/uncategorized/ableism

Stramondo, Joseph A. 2020. "COVID-19 Traige and Disability: What NOT To Do." *Bioethics Today*, March 30, 2020. https://bioethicstoday.org/blog/covid-19-triage-and-disability-what-not-to-do/

The Arc. 2020a. "Disability Discrimination Complaint Filed Over COVID-19 Treatment Rationing Plan in Washington State." *The Arc*, March 23, 2020. https://thearc.org/blog/disability-discrimination-complaint-filed-over-covid-19-treatment-rationing-plan-in-washington-state/

The Arc. 2020b. "HHS-OCR Complaints Re COVID-19 Medical Discrimination." *The Arc*, March 23, 2020. https://thearc.org/resource/hhs-ocr-complaint-of-disability-rights-washington-self-advocates-in-leadership-the-arc-of-the-united-states-and-ivanova-smith/

Tilley, Elizabeth, Jan Walmsley, Sarah Earle, and Dorothy Atkinson. 2012. "'The Silence Is Roaring': Sterilization, Reproductive Rights and Women with Intellectual Disabilities." *Disability & Society* 27 (3): 413–426.

Tolchin, Benjamin, Sarah C. Hull, and Katherine Kraschel. 2021. "Triage and Justice in an Unjust Pandemic: Ethical Allocation of Scarce Medical Resources in the Setting of Racial and Socioeconomic Disparities." *Journal of Medical Ethics* 47 (3): 200–202.

U.S. Department of Health and Human Services. 2020a. "OCR Resolves Civil Rights Complaint Against Pennsylvania After It Revises Its Pandemic Health Care Triaging Policies to Protect Against Disability Discrimination." *Department of Health and Human Services*, April 16, 2020. https://www.hhs.gov/about/news/2020/04/16/ocr-resolves-civil-rights-complaint-against-pennsylvania-after-it-revises-its-pandemic-health-care.html

U.S. Department of Health and Human Services. 2020b. "OCR Resolves Complaint with Tennessee After It Revises Its Triage Plans to Protect Against Disability Discrimination." *Department of Health and Human Services*, June 26, 2020. https://www.hhs.gov/about/news/2020/06/26/ocr-resolves-complaint-tennessee-after-it-revises-its-triage-plans-protect-against-disability.html

U.S. National Council on Disability. 2019. *Medical Futility and Disabilty Bias*. Washington, DC: National Council on Disability. https://www.ncd.gov/report/medical-futility-and-disability-bias/

U.S. National Council on Disability. 2021. *2021 Progress Report: The Impact of COVID-19 on People with Disabilities*. Washington, DC: National Council on Disability. https://www.ncd.gov/report/an-extra/

United Nations. 2020 *Policy Brief: A Disability-Inclusive Response to COVID-19*. United Nations. https://www.un.org/sites/un2.un.org/files/2020/05/sg_policy_brief_on_persons_with_disabilities_final.pdf

Wasserman, David T., and Adrienne Asch. 2005. "Where Is the Sin in Synecdoche? Prenatal Testing and the Parent-Child Relationship." In *Quality of Life and Human Difference Genetic Testing, Health*

Care, and Disability, edited by David Wasserman, Jerome Bickenbach, and Robert Wachbroit, pp. 172–216. Cambridge: Cambridge University Press.

White, Douglas B., and Bernard Lo. 2021. "Mitigating Inequities and Saving Lives with ICU Triage during the COVID-19 Pandemic." *American Journal of Respiratory and Critical Care Medicine* 203 (3): 287–295. https://doi.org/10.1164/rccm.202010-3809CP

White, Douglas B., Lisa Villarroel, and John L. Hick. 2021. "Inequitable Access to Hospital Care—Protecting Disadvantaged Populations during Public Health Emergencies." *New England Journal of Medicine* 385 (24): 2211–2214.

Yong, Ed. 2020. "How the Pandemic Will End." *The Atlantic*, March 25, 2020. https://www.theatlantic.com/health/archive/2020/03/how-will-coronavirus-end/608719

2

INCORPORATING SOCIAL DETERMINANTS OF HEALTH INTO CRISIS STANDARDS OF CARE

April Dworetz

The necessity of resource allocation and the development of Crisis Standards of Care (CSC) in the COVID-19 pandemic raised ethical questions regarding who would receive the potentially beneficial treatment (Rajczi et al. 2021; Emanuel et al. 2020). The goal, to apportion such scarce resources fairly, requires the balancing of numerous ethical concerns to generate an equitable rationing scheme. Who should get the resources? How should they be apportioned? Who should make the decisions? What criteria should CSC include? Do exclusion criteria perpetuate bias? How do we compensate for structural racism and ableism? No one ethical principle is sufficient for a fair resource allocation system. But the process of developing these CSC must meet specific ethical guidelines.

I propose that to follow ethical guidelines, CSC developers should directly address ableism and other discriminatory practices that affect well-being. In this chapter, I review aspects of the social determinants of health (SDH). and their incorporation into Crisis Standards of Care. Though I discuss socioeconomic status, I focus on disabled people and people of color. Specific adjustments to the criteria for CSC can make allocations fairer, but justice requires a more explicit method of addressing the systemic inequities for disabled people and other groups of marginalized patients. I endorse including a marker for SDH in the criteria that determine who receives rationed resources (NASEM 2020; Laventhal et al. 2020; Emanuel et al. 2020; Scheunemann and White 2011; Persad et al. 2009; White et al. 2009; White and Lo 2020).

Ableism, Racism, and the Social Determinants of Health

Even before the COVID-19 pandemic, The Institute of Medicine (now part of the National Academy of Medicine) Committee on Guidance for Establishing Standards of Care for Use in Disaster Situations provided direction for establishing CSC (Institute of Medicine [IOM] 2010). They claimed that such medical care should not deviate from ethical norms despite limiting treatment for a subset of patients (Scheunemann and White 2011; NASEM 2012; Daniels and Sabin 1997). To do this, CSC developers should base rationing decisions on ethical principles, including fairness, transparency, and accountability (IOM 2010; Baum et al. 2009; Laventhal et al. 2020). Fairness requires righting the wrongs of disparities in healthcare

DOI: 10.4324/9781003502623-4

due to racism, classism, and ableism. Transparent and accountable processes promote medical trust, something often missing for people with disabilities and other marginalized and oppressed groups. Consistency and proportionality allow for fair practices in triage. With this endorsement, the Institute of Medicine set the stage for ethically derived CSC.

Ethical considerations have grounded many of the nation's CSC. Until civil rights and disability groups addressed ageism, racism, and ableism in CSC, some of the concerns for older people, people of color, and people with disabilities did not appear in the discussion. These groups challenged some of the ethical principles used to develop CSC that introduced injustice. They broached the issue of the SDH. Most of the CSC that were developed prior to or early in the COVID-19 pandemic did not take into consideration the SDH (White and Lo 2021, 2022; Cleveland Manchanda et al. 2021). A few changed with the input of the racial equity and disability advocacy groups who raised the issue. In this chapter I discuss the issues that arise from racism, classism, and ableism in terms of SDH and CSC. But I concentrate on people of color and people with disabilities because of the intersection with poverty, and because developers of CSC can affect inequity most by amending the criteria for rationing of scarce resources for people of color and people with disabilities.

SDH negatively influence people living in poverty, people of color, and people with disabilities. The baseline elements associated with SDH include congested housing, stability of housing, access to healthy foods, unsafe environments restricting exercise, jobs requiring more contact with others, need to use public transportation, worse education, immigration status, poor healthcare access, experience of bias while receiving healthcare, higher rates of chronic disease, and greater exposure to pollution (Cleveland Manchanda et al. 2020; Tai et al. 2021; Emerson et al. 2011; Persad 2021; Rollston and Galea 2020; Sabatello et al. 2020; Schmidt et al. 2022). These factors adversely affect health outcomes and increase health disparities. People thus affected are placed at a disadvantage when being triaged.

Health disparities or inequities worsen health consequences due to preventable social, economic, and environmental hardships (Krahn et al. 2015, S198). As with all people subject to negative SDH, people with disabilities have worse health outcomes than people without disabilities (Emerson et al. 2011). To clarify, depending on their disability, disabled people do not always live with poor health. And disability itself does not necessarily negatively impact health outcomes. That is, poor health outcomes may not relate to the underlying disability, but likely have to do with social determinants (Krahn et al. 2015; Iezzoni et al. 2021). The discrimination and inequity that occur in terms of disparities in healthcare for people with disabilities result in "unhealthier lifestyle behaviors and poorer mental health, creating a cycle of more chronic conditions, poorer health, and increasing functional limitations" (Krahn et al. 2015, S202). Studies show that compared with people without disabilities, those with disabilities were more likely to experience a greater burden of chronic disease, breast and lung cancer, and higher mortality rates (Iezzoni 2011). In addition, Black, Latinx, and Indigenous people are more likely to have chronic diseases such as hypertension, diabetes, and heart disease due to SDH. These chronic diseases, in turn, increase the risk of worse outcomes, including higher mortality, from COVID-19 infection (Bambra et al. 2020).

For people with disabilities, the poor health outcomes associated with SDH must be distinguished from the health outcomes, if any, associated with their disability. In relation to this, Jackie Leach Scully argues that there are three assumptions that "critically endanger the rights of people with disability in a situation of pandemic triage" (Scully 2020, 212). These assumptions include health status related to the disability, quality of life conjectures, and notions of social utility. Though the public, generally, and healthcare professionals, specifically, may make these suppositions, many people with disabilities have good health status, enjoyable quality of life, and social utility. This distinction is particularly important when evaluating a patient for triage inclusion criteria. Instead of expectations, individual assessment of each patient for chances of recovery from COVID-19 creates a more just criterion.

In times of crisis, discrimination can worsen for marginalized communities (Sabatello et al. 2020). For example, during the COVID-19 pandemic, people with disabilities living in nursing homes and group homes had higher infectivity and mortality from COVID-19 (Andrews et al. 2021; Guidry-Grimes et al. 2020). The overcrowding in these homes made social distancing difficult (Landes et al. 2022). People with disabilities who required multiple aides for personal care had increased exposure to COVID-19. People with certain communication-based and cognitive disabilities may not have understood information presented inaccessibly. Expectedly, the failure of healthcare professionals and institutions to accommodate people with disabilities so that they could comprehend instructions or treatment choices created further medical problems for people with disabilities. Patients with intellectual or developmental disabilities, particularly Down syndrome and cerebral palsy, have higher mortality due to COVID-19 than people without disabilities (Landes et al. 2022; Turk et al. 2020).

For people whose negative health outcomes result from social dynamics, neglecting SDH fails to treat them with equity. These factors provide a rationale to adjust CSC for marginalized persons. A proactive development process that prevents disability, race, ethnic, and socioeconomic discrimination will go far to create unbiased and well-grounded CSC.

Ableism and Racism in Healthcare and Crisis Standards of Care

Ableism is a complicated concept and thus defies an easy definition. One characterization refers to judgmental attitudes and behaviors causing discrimination toward people with disabilities, whether physical, psychological, or intellectual (Smith 2023). Another description proposes that disability bias and stigma create ableism (Barnes 2016). But according to David M. Pena-Guzman and Joel Michael Reynolds, ableism extends beyond the issue of bias and stigma to the use of perceptions of normalcy that determine "the quality, meaning, value, and differences of human life through the lens of abilities and ability expectations" (Peña-Guzman and Reynolds 2019, 215). In this chapter, I use an amalgam of these explanations of ableism to apply to clinical practice. This definition suggests that viewing people with disabilities via ability and normality perspectives creates erroneous judgments.

Healthcare professionals and bioethicists often use the concepts of ability and normality to attribute negative attitudes toward people with disabilities, causing harm in healthcare (Reynolds 2018; Peña-Guzman and Reynolds 2019). There are important analogies and intersections between ableism and racism on this point. Camara Jones describes that personally mediated actions, internalized values, or structural grounds whether intentional or not can trigger racism (Jones 2000). These same factors apply to the development of ableism.[1] In a 2021 study of physicians' attitudes toward people with disabilities, Lisa I. Iezzoni and colleagues found that "large proportions of practicing US physicians might hold biased or stigmatized perceptions of people with disabilities" (Iezzoni et al. 2021, 301). Peña-Guzmán and Reynolds claim that healthcare professionals exhibit implicit disability bias which results in "epistemic ignorance about disability" (Peña-Guzman and Reynolds 2019, 216). This lack of knowledge about disability causes healthcare professionals both to stay unaware of the lived experiences of people with different types of disabilities despite claims to the contrary and to fail to acknowledge the expertise of people with disabilities "as experts about their own experiences and that of their communities" (Peña-Guzman and Reynolds 2019, 216). In addition, a poor understanding of disability and assumptions about the quality of life, especially when compared to "normality" can influence treatment choices and outcomes (Andrews et al. 2021; Iezzoni et al. 2021; Scully 2020).

On a larger scale, healthcare institutions have policies and physical environments that perpetrate structural ableism. Examples of systemic disability discrimination include inaccessible clinical environments in which exam tables, mammography and other radiology machines, weight scales, and communication strategies are not designed for people with mobility, sensory, or intellectual/developmental disabilities (Sabatello et al. 2020; Iezzoni 2011). Explicit and implicit biases by healthcare professionals as well as structural ableism not only create unjust conditions but may result in inequitable provision of healthcare, especially when deciding who gets scarce resources.

Racism and classism, embedded in the healthcare system and triggering inequities of health, also exacerbate injustice when not addressed in CSC (Cleveland Manchanda et al. 2020; Rollston and Galea 2020; Schmidt, Gostin, and Williams 2020; Schmidt, Shaikh, Sadecki, Buttenheim, et al. 2022; Schmidt, Roberts and Eneanya 2022; Tai et al. 2021; White and Lo 2021; Yancy 2020). Of even greater concern is when racism and classicism intersect with ableism. Racial and ethnic minority people are more likely than White people to experience disability. The connection of racial or ethnic minority and disability results in a higher rate of socially based healthcare disparities. In an interview with George Yancy, Talila A. Lewis detailed an explanation of this connection (Lewis 2023). Lewis argues that ableism involves racism, sexism, capitalism, and disability. Lewis further claims that "ableism plays a leading role in how we frame, understand, construct, and respond to race, class, gender, sexual orientation, ethnicity, nationality, criminal status, disability, and countless other identities. Meaning, not only is ableism central to the construction of what people think disability is, but ableism frames every other marginalized identity as well." (Lewis 2023).

The intersection of people who are subject to SDH places people with disability in a particularly vulnerable position. Importantly, Lewis asserts that the different communities experiencing these harms must stick together to fight oppression: "[a]nti-Black racism and dis/ableism must be understood, addressed and dismantled in relation to each other (simultaneously)." (Lewis 2023). These actions, applying to all persons at risk for SDH, must occur when determining resource allocation in times of scarcity.

Prior to public input in CSC, healthcare professionals and bioethicists did not make allowances for the groups of patients who experience SDH (Ne'eman et al. 2021). Disability and civil rights advocates, scholars, and organizations have endorsed adjusting for discrimination against people with disabilities and people of color (Brown and Goodwin 2020; Cleveland Manchanda et al. 2020; Guidry-Grimes et al. 2020; Hick et al. 2021; Mello et al. 2020; Persad 2021; Schmidt, Roberts, and Eneanya 2022; White and Lo 2021, 2022). They recommended factoring the SDH into resource allocation protocols. This important modification supports people with disability, people of color, and people living in poverty. It at least partially corrects for SDH that previously had not been included in CSC. By representing neighborhoods in terms of disadvantage, two instruments have been developed to indirectly gauge SDH: the Social Vulnerability Index and Area Deprivation Index (Hu et al. 2018). These indices evaluate employment, education, and environmental characteristics to denote area deprivation. They reflect not only disadvantage but also health outcomes.

Not all developers of CSC agree that they should correct for existing inequities (Prusak et al. 2021). However, by ignoring the SDH, people of color and people with disabilities are *once again* discriminated against (Schmidt, Roberts, and Eneanya 2022; Sabatello et al. 2020; Tai et al. 2021; Rollston and Galea 2020). Neglecting SDH fails to treat as equals people whose negative health outcomes result from oppressive social dynamics and healthcare practices. Although saving the greatest number of people is the major target of CSC, correcting injustice applies to CSC goals. The Institute of Medicine emphasizes the importance of both fairness and justice as ethical principles in the development and implementation of CSC (IOM 2010; Hick et al. 2021). From the principle of fairness, it follows that CSC must adjust for the effects of racism, classicism, and ableism, among other interpersonally and structurally inequitable features of social life. The National Academies of Science, Engineering and Medicine also agrees with the goal of creating CSC that combat injustice (NASEM 2020). I have argued that this should be done, but how one most effectively integrates components that adjust for healthcare disparities into the policies that outline scarce resource allocation remains to be determined.

Disability, Race, and Ethical Issues in Developing Crisis Standards of Care

The recognition of the SDH affecting COVID-19 survival and the advocacy of disability and civil rights groups triggered the examination of some of the ethical guidelines for developing CSC. The ethical principles of justice, beneficence, and nonmaleficence take on a new perspective when viewed through the eyes of disability and civil rights advocates. This section reviews these arguments.

As an example of revised ethical guidelines that addressed these concerns, Michelle Mello and colleagues proposed six recommendations regarding the protection of disability rights when drawing up CSC (Mello et al. 2020):

- Including disability rights advocates in the development of CSC
- Prohibiting the use of exclusion criteria and quality of life factors
- Utilizing scores for the potential for hospital survival, but not long-term survival
- Banning private home-use ventilator redistribution
- Creating a triage team to make triage decisions for the hospital and training the triage team regarding disability rights.

I expand upon these suggestions in the rest of this section.

Including Disability Rights Advocates in the Development of CSC

In 2010, the Institute of Medicine suggested engagement with "the public and stakeholders" while developing CSC (IOM 2010). Laura Guidry-Grimes and colleagues, taking this a step further, called for community engagement in CSC development that includes groups having insight into the intersectional nature of disability (Guidry-Grimes et al. 2020). This guidance allowed for the interested parties to provide their unique viewpoints during the development of CSC. Individual disability activists who represented a more intersectional aspect of the community and disability organizations created public advocacy groups (Andrews et al. 2021). These alliances provided information to CSC developers and made sure that meetings offered necessary accommodations such as American Sign Language interpreters, captioning, and lay language so that the disability community could receive information about triage possibilities. The process is intended to be an iterative activity requiring communication and education in both directions between CSC creators and the community.

These disability advocacy groups pushed for eliminating ableism and other discriminatory actions in CSC criteria. In California, for example, a group of disability activists wrote to the governor and the secretary of the Health and Human Services Agency in California objecting to a lack of input from disability advocacy groups during the development of the state's CSC (Center 2020). The letter's authors advocated for the inclusion of a statement that requires protection from discrimination toward people with disabilities (Center 2020, 2). These safeguards included addressing the "barriers that routinely subject disabled people to less effective care" and educating triage teams about communities of patients that often experience discrimination in healthcare (Center 2020, 3).

In addition to these recommendations from California, disability rights groups across the country lodged complaints of disability discrimination with the U.S. Department of Health and Human Services (HHS) Office for Civil Rights (OCR) about government resource allocation guidelines. The OCR received a multitude of grievances and reviewed lawsuits regarding discrimination against people with disabilities in state or institutional CSC (Savin 2020). In response, they put out an advisory letter reviewing the legal requirements to comply with the civil rights of patients, including patients with disabilities (Action 2020). HHS clarified that "civil rights protections remain in full force and effect during disasters or emergencies including the COVID-19 pandemic" (Office of Civil Rights [OCR] 2022, 1). Furthermore, HHS enforced laws that prohibit discrimination on the basis of disability as detailed in Section 504 of the Rehabilitation Act Section 1557 of the Affordable Care Act. In forming CSC, the HHS instructed that those who make decisions about triage "must analyze the specific patient's ability to benefit from the treatment sought, free from stereotypes and bias about disability, including prejudicial preconceptions and assessments of quality of life, or judgments about a person's relative 'worth' based on the presence or absence of disabilities" (OCR 2022, 3). Throughout the COVID-19 pandemic, the OCR insisted on revisions of several CSC due to complaints regarding the incorporation of discriminatory criteria (Mello et al. 2020; OCR 2022).

Rejecting Categorical Exclusions

Disability advocacy groups and the Department of Health and Human Services rejected the use of categorical exclusions, which bar patients from any eligibility for scarce resources, in triage decisions because they promote injustice (Ne'eman et al. 2021; Solomon et al. 2020; White and Lo 2020). For example, categorical exclusion of all patients with a specific disability has the potential to exclude from triage people with disability who experience a better quality of life and have greater potential for survival than some people without disability (Yancy 2020). To exclude them categorically, which is to say, based on disability, from getting limited resources would introduce ableism. The same goes for age exclusions. Some older people may have a higher rate of survival than some younger people. To exclude them categorically from getting limited resources would introduce age bias. Though many state CSC proposals initially included categorical exclusions, many ethicists deemed their use in CSC unethical (Auriemma et al. 2020; Mello et al. 2020; NAM 2020). Making all patients eligible and then factoring in relevant and specific criteria to determine which patients are likeliest to survive is preferable to categorical exclusions. Evaluation of the *individual* patient in terms of survival from the acute illness generates a more just process and should guide triage decisions (Guidry-Grimes et al. 2020).

The law compels a personal evaluation before excluding an individual with disability from assistance or a program (Ne'eman et al. 2021; 835). That is, the law makes categorical exclusions illegal. The HHS Office for Civil Rights explicitly disallowed the use of categorical exclusions of disability for CSC (OCR 2022). One example is the Alabama CSC that categorically excluded patients with "severe or profound mental retardation." (Mello et al. 2020, e26(1); Andrews et al. 2021). In another case, the state of Tennessee's CSC categorically excluded people with spinal muscular atrophy, a disorder sometimes requiring a ventilator to help with breathing. The OCR rejected these exclusions and required revision to the CSC. The criteria for CSC triage may include these factors as one of many or employ them as tiebreakers (Auriemma et al. 2020; NASEM 2020; NAM 2020).

Omitting Quality of Life Considerations

Disability advocacy groups also recommended omitting quality of life evaluations as part of the criteria for the allocation of scarce resources (Ne'eman et al. 2021; White and Lo 2020; Sabatello et al. 2020; Mello et al. 2020; Solomon et al. 2020). As discussed previously, healthcare professionals often rate the quality of life of people with disabilities as worse than the people with disabilities rate their own quality of life despite decades of social science research demonstrating that disabled people experience similar levels of quality of life (Iezzoni et al. 2021; Basnet 2001). Many people without disabilities tend to see disability from negative perspectives, not from the lived experiences of people with disabilities. The quality of life of people with disabilities typically depends more on the SDH than on the disability (Andrews et al. 2021). "A disabled person's ability to achieve their goals depends less on the nature of disability and individual coping skills than on personal, familial, and systemic interactions with schools, employers, healthcare providers and communities" (Andrews et al. 2021, 457). Such findings suggest that including quality of life in CSC criteria would give authority to false, prejudicial assumptions about people with disabilities.

Rejecting Scores for Long-Term Survival

Disability advocates also suggested that guidelines for the allocation of scarce resources exclude life expectancy, long-term survival, and life-years (Ne'eman et al. 2021; Solomon et al. 2020). Instead, they recommended using short-term (to discharge, six months, or, at a maximum, one year). survival as one of the CSC guidelines. Long-term survival is inequitable regarding disability and age (Center 2020). Healthcare professionals have difficulty making accurate and valid prognoses especially for diseases or disorders that are not well-researched and for prognoses based on old data. Long-term survival may also incorporate implicit bias and, therefore, erroneous prognoses (Sabatello et al. 2020). Even if long-term survival could be estimated, it does not address the SDH that affect people with disabilities, people of color, and other marginalized groups (Cleveland Manchanda et al. 2020; Ne'eman et al. 2021; White and Lo 2021) sing long-term survival compounds these health inequities. As a result of this concern, including prognosis of only up to six months or one year fits into the utilitarian goal of saving the most people, whilst it also respects people affected by the SDH.

Equity Problems with Determining Short-Term Survival

Most CSC use the Sequential Organ Failure Assessment (SOFA). scale or the modified SOFA scale to evaluate the likelihood of survival from COVID-19 (Biddison et al. 2019; White and Lo 2020; White and Lo 2021; Tolchin et al. 2021; Antommaria et al. 2020). The SOFA scale, a validated system for predicting mortality due to sepsis, a bacterial infection of the blood, uses multiple measurements of organ dysfunction to predict mortality in critically ill adult patients (Ferreira et al. 2001; Sanchez-Pinto et al. 2021). But SOFA scores do not predict short-term mortality for COVID-19 (Maves et al. 2020).

Applying SOFA and modified SOFA generates major ethical problems. Higher scores (worse scores leading to less likelihood of receiving scarce resources) often affect people with disabilities and Black patients and have nothing to do with their potential for death due to COVID-19 (Center 2020; Ne'eman et al. 2021). Thus, SOFA scores may discriminate against some patients with disabilities and Black patients (Andrews et al. 2021; Guidry-Grimes et al. 2020; Miller et al. 2021; Tolchin et al. 2021). One way SOFA discriminates against people with disabilities is through the use of the Glasgow Coma Scale, a section of SOFA (Guidry-Grimes et al. 2020; Ne'eman et al. 2021; Cleveland Manchanda et al. 2020; Fins 2021). Developed for patients at varying levels of consciousness, the Glasgow Coma Scale adds points for patients with unintelligible speech, thus worsening the chance for resources. Patients with a speech disability due to a movement disorder, for example, will get a worse SOFA score even though their disability does not worsen their prognosis. In addition, the Glasgow Coma Scale inappropriately assesses and potentially discriminates against people in a minimally conscious state due to traumatic brain injury (Fins 2021). To remedy these disadvantages and to comply legally with requiring adjustments for people with disabilities, disability groups recommended modifications of the SOFA scores COVID-19 patients with disabilities (OCR 2022).

Besides people with disabilities, Black patients also have adverse scores using SOFA (Cleveland Manchanda et al. 2020; Miller et al. 2021; Tolchin et al. 2021; Schmidt, Roberts, and Eneanya 2022). In a study by Miller and colleagues, Black patients have a lower rate of mortality than White patients with the same SOFA scores (Miller et al. 2021). This means that a Black patient with the same SOFA score as a White patient has a higher chance of survival, but their triage categories are the same. One commonly cited cause for unfair SOFA scores due to race is creatinine levels. Due to the physical effects of structural racism, these levels are typically higher in Black people than White people despite equivalent kidney function (Ne'eman et al. 2021; White and Lo 2021; Diao et al. 2021; Schmidt, Roberts, and Eneanya 2022). In addition, higher SOFA scores may be due to more severe illness in Black patients with COVID-19 because of health disparities (Cleveland Manchanda et al. 2020: Miller et al. 2021; Schmidt, Roberts, and Eneanya 2022; Tolchin et al. 2021). Higher scores may also occur because Black patients may be sicker at the time of presentation (Tolchin et al. 2021). The many SDH including less education about COVID-19, less economic stability, and less access to healthcare in some Black communities may have caused some Black patients to present when more ill than White people (Bambra et al. 2020). This suggests that using SOFA scores as part of triage guidelines exacerbates healthcare inequities and puts Black patients at a disadvantage in obtaining scarce resources.

Moreover, SOFA scores do not reliably predict outcome from COVID-19 infection. As mentioned above, they were originally developed for estimating survival from sepsis. In a study evaluating SOFA scores and mortality due to COVID-19 pneumonia requiring mechanical ventilation, the SOFA score poorly predicted mortality (Raschke et al. 2021). In another study, most of the patients who scored highest on SOFA or MSOFA survived (Grissom et al. 2010). Though SOFA or MSOFA scores may not correlate to mortality from COVID-19 infection, an accurate predictive scoring system does not exist, and so CSC developers have chosen the best and easiest score they have available (White et al. 2009).

More research and a better system for the prediction of short-term mortality due to COVID-19 infection is needed. Schmidt and colleagues have suggested dropping the SOFA score altogether or modifying the SOFA score to account for the discrimination caused by the Glasgow Coma Scale and creatinine scores (Schmidt, Roberts, and Eneanya 2022). Given that a replacement scoring system has not been developed and SOFA may promote systemic racism and ableism, a supplementary scoring measure such as the area deprivation index described earlier in the chapter should be added to help balance such discrimination (White and Lo 2022; Tolchin et al. 2021; Schmidt, Roberts, and Eneanya 2022; Miller et al. 2021).

Balancing Ethical Principles to Make CSC More Equitable

White and Lo, who amended their original CSC protocol by adding the area deprivation index, initially developed a CSC known as the Pittsburgh protocol soon after the COVID-19 pandemic began (White and Lo 2021, 2020). Until they read critiques about their CSC using long-term prognosis and ignoring structural inequities of healthcare, they failed to realize that their strategy ignored such injustice (Schmidt, Roberts, and Eneanya 2022). As a result of this criticism, White and Lo went back to the ethical drawing board and revised their primary ethical goals. They suggested that using the utilitarian theory of saving the most lives for CSC would promote discrimination and result in overall harm to society (White and Lo 2021, 288-9). To prevent this harm, they added the public health goal of improving "the aggregate health outcomes of populations" by addressing biases for their criteria for rationing of healthcare (White and Lo 2021, 290). They reshaped their CSC to incorporate issues of justice, including changing the criteria of long-term survival from five years to one year (many disability bioethicists, researchers, and advocates argued for six months or survival to discharge). They attempted to alleviate the inequity due to SDH for patients living in areas of socioeconomic disadvantage by using the area deprivation index and therefore decreasing the overall CSC score. The lower score would give the patient a better chance to receive scarce resources such as a ventilator or ICU bed.

Keeping Home Ventilators with their Owners

Besides correcting for SDH, disability advocacy groups also suggested not reallocating patients' personal ventilators when hospitalized with COVID-19 (Center 2020; Ne'eman et al. 2021; Reynolds et al. 2021). New York's CSC initially incorporated the possibility of excluding patients with their own ventilators from triage and reallocating these home ventilators to other patients. This criterion was disallowed by the OCR and sent back for revision. Reynolds and colleagues also formed a moral argument against reallocating personal ventilators. They contended that the personal ventilator is an "integrated technology," vital to the owner's functioning for the long term, and part of their "relational narrative identity" (Reynolds et al. 2021, 275). That is, a personal ventilator is an extension of the owner's body for which reallocation is similar to amputation of a body part without consent, making forced reallocation unethical. In a similar vein, CSC should not triage by resource intensity or duration of need.

The National Academy of Medicine stated that requiring more resources is not an indication to lower the chances of receiving scarce treatment due to disability or age (NAM 2020).

Triage Teams

Many CSC recommended that a triage team make determinations about who receives scarce resources (Antommaria et al. 2020; Andrews et al. 2021; Brown and Goodwin 2020; Guidry-Grimes et al. 2020; NASEM 2020; UC Critical Care 2020; White and Lo 2021). A pre-selected team or teams would implement triage so that individual healthcare professionals at the bed-side, who have a direct and overriding responsibility to their individual patients, do not make rationing decisions. In response to concerns that the triage teams could be subject to implicit bias, disability scholars have suggested deleting immaterial patient characteristics such as race, disability, or insurance status; ensuring diversity of the triage team; training the triage team regarding implicit bias specifically about race, ethnicity, and disability; and making triage teams aware of ways to manage triage scores if they are biased (Cleveland Manchanda et al. 2020; Schmidt, Roberts, and Eneanya 2022; Mello et al. 2020; Brown and Goodwin 2020; Hick et al. 2021; Savin 2020). Appropriate advocates would train the teams to recognize disability and racial discrimination and hold each member of the team accountable. People of racial, ethnic, and disability diversity would represent the teams. In addition, the teams would be made up of people who have clinical experience with people with disabilities (Sabatello et al. 2020; White and Lo 2020). Finally, fair triage appeal processes would address *post hoc* concerns about discrimination.

Conclusion

Although the revisions of The Pittsburgh Protocol and a few other CSC exemplified substantial gains by disability and civil rights advocates, the CSC were not built upon a foundation of disability and racial justice, which is to say, they were geared toward neither fairness, nor equality, nor equity. Our society, as well as our medical system, has a long way to go before we achieve racial and disability justice. While imperfect and contested, debates over CSC development made progress toward a shared vision that in fact prioritizes such justice.

The development and revision of CSC, especially those written later in the pandemic after the activists and scholars articulated their perspectives, benefited immensely from recommendations by disability and racial justice groups. The legal impetus from the Office for Civil Rights aided these groups in initiating many of these changes. In this chapter, I described multiple insights and actionable items that participant advocates and ethicists have argued for. These include:

- Rejecting categorical exclusions,
- Preventing quality of life inclusions,
- Limiting long-term prognoses as criteria to a maximum of one year or less (with strong argument for survival to discharge),
- Including individual modifications to SOFA scores that actively mitigate racial and disability-based bias,
- Disallowing reallocation of personal ventilators,
- Prohibiting assessment of resource intensity,

- Incorporating racial and disability awareness and education in triage teams,
- Adding proxies for social determinates of health such as the Social Vulnerability Index
- Developing less racist and ableist scoring instruments for determining survival from COVID-19 infection.

Each of these ethical considerations considers the SDH, a necessary consideration for equitable CSC. These ethical factors were included in some CSC thanks to response from and engagement with disability and racial advocates. Such positive changes suggest that public policy scholars sometimes hear and respond to the stakeholders' call for justice. Such sustained involvement with stakeholders, especially and specifically from those who are a part of historically marginalized communities, will continue to improve policy, not just for CSC, but for all healthcare policy.

Note

1 Personally mediated actions of ableism are experienced at the individual, interpersonal level by disabled people. Internalized ableism explains the negative attitudes of people toward disabled people. And structural ableism stems from institutional policies that limit healthcare to disabled people.

Work Cited

Andrews, E. E., K.B. Ayers, K.S. Brown, D.S. Dunn. 2021. "No Body is Expendable: Medical Rationing and Disability Justice During the COVID-19 Pandemic." *American Psychologist* 76 (3): 451–461.

Antommaria, A. H. M., T. S. Gibb, A. L. McGuire, P. R. Wolpe, M. K. Wynia, M. K. Applewhite, A. Caplan, D. S. Diekema, D. M. Hester, L. S. Lehmann, R. McLeod-Sordjan, T. Schiff, H. K. Tabor, S. E. Wieten, J. T. Eberl, and Directors Task Force of the Association of Bioethics Program. 2020. "Ventilator Triage Policies During the COVID-19 Pandemic at U.S. Hospitals Associated with Members of the Association of Bioethics Program Directors." *Annals of Intern Medicine* 173 (3): 188–194. https://doi.org/10.7326/M20-1738

Auriemma, C. L., A. M. Molinero, A. J. Houtrow, G. Persad, D. B. White, and S. D. Halpern. 2020. "Eliminating Categorical Exclusion Criteria in Crisis Standards of Care Frameworks." *American Journal of Bioethics* 20 (7): 28–36. https://doi.org/10.1080/15265161.2020.1764141

Bambra, C., R. Riordan, J. Ford, and F. Matthews. 2020. "The COVID-19 pandemic and health inequalities." *J Epidemiol Community Health* 74 (11): 964–968. https://doi.org/10.1136/jech-2020-214401

Barnes, Elizabeth. 2016. *The Minority Body.* New York: Oxford University Press.

Basnet, I. 2001. "Health Care Professionals and their Attitudes toward and Decisions Affecting Disabled People." In *Handbook of Disability Studies*, edited by Katherine D. Seelman, Gary L. Albrecht, and Michael Bury, 450–467. London: Sage Publications.

Baum, N. M., P. D. Jacobson, and S. D. Goold. 2009. ""Listen to the people": public deliberation about social distancing measures in a pandemic." *American Journal of Bioethics* 9 (11): 4–14. https://doi.org/10.1080/15265160903197531

Biddison, E. Lee Daugherty, Ruth Faden, Howard S. Gwon, Darren P. Mareiniss, Alan C. Regenberg, Monica Schoch-Spana, Jack Schwartz, and Eric S. Toner. 2019. "Too Many Patients…A Framework to Guide Statewide Allocation of Scarce Mechanical Ventilation During Disasters." *Chest* 155 (4): 848–854. https://doi.org/10.1016/j.chest.2018.09.025

Brown, M. J., and J. Goodwin. 2020. "Allocating Medical Resources in the Time of COVID-19." *New England Journal of Medicine* 382 (22): e79. https://doi.org/10.1056/NEJMc2009666

Center for the Disability Rights Education and Defense Fund. 2020. "California Organizations Letter re Healthcare Rationing to Governor Newsom and Secretary Ghaly."

Cleveland Manchanda, E. C., C. Sanky, and J. M. Appel. 2021. "Crisis Standards of Care in the USA: A Systematic Review and Implications for Equity Amidst COVID-19." *Journal of Racial and Ethnic Health Disparities* 8 (4): 824–836. https://doi.org/10.1007/s40615-020-00840-5

Cleveland Manchanda, E., C. Couillard, and K. Sivashanker. 2020. "Inequity in Crisis Standards of Care." *The New England Journal of Medicine* 383 (4): e16. https://doi.org/10.1056/NEJMp2011359

Daniels, N., and J. Sabin. 1997. "Limits to health care: fair procedures, democratic deliberation, and the legitimacy problem for insurers." *Philosophy and Public Affairs* 26 (4): 303–350. https://doi.org/10.1111/j.1088-4963.1997.tb00082.x

Diao, J. A., L. A. Inker, A. S. Levey, H. Tighiouart, N. R. Powe, and A. K. Manrai. 2021. "In Search of a Better Equation - Performance and Equity in Estimates of Kidney Function." *The New England Journal of Medicine* 384 (5): 396–399. https://doi.org/10.1056/NEJMp2028243

Emanuel, E. J., G. Persad, R. Upshur, B. Thome, M. Parker, A. Glickman, C. Zhang, C. Boyle, M. Smith, and J. P. Phillips. 2020. "Fair Allocation of Scarce Medical Resources in the Time of COVID-19." *The New England Journal of Medicine* 382 (21): 2049–2055. https://doi.org/10.1056/NEJMsb2005114

Emerson, E., R. Madden, H. Graham, G. Llewellyn, C. Hatton, and J. Robertson. 2011. "The Health of Disabled People and the Social Determinants of Health." *Public Health* 125 (3): 145–47. https://doi.org/10.1016/j.puhe.2010.11.003

Ferreira, F. L., D. P. Bota, A. Bross, C. Melot, and J. L. Vincent. 2001. "Serial Evaluation of the SOFA Score to Predict Outcome in Critically Ill Patients." *JAMA* 286 (14): 1754–1758. https://doi.org/10.1001/jama.286.14.1754

Fins, J. J. 2021. "Disorders of Consciousness, Disability Rights and Triage During the COVID-19 Pandemic: Even the Best of Intentions Can Lead to Bias." *The Journal of Philosophy of Disability* 1: 211–229. https://doi.org/10.5840/jpd20218174

Grissom, C. K., S. M. Brown, K. G. Kuttler, J. P. Boltax, J. Jones, A. R. Jephson, and J. F. Orme, Jr. 2010. "A Modified Sequential Organ Failure Assessment Score for Critical Care Triage." *Disaster Medicine and Public Health Preparedness* 4 (4): 277–284. https://doi.org/10.1001/dmp.2010.40

Guidry-Grimes, L., K. Savin, J. A. Stramondo, J. M. Reynolds, M. Tsaplina, T. B. Burke, A. Ballantyne, E. F. Kittay, D. Stahl, J. L. Scully, R. Garland-Thomson, A. Tarzian, D. Dorfman, and J. J. Fins. 2020. "Disability Rights as a Necessary Framework for Crisis Standards of Care and the Future of Health Care." *Hastings Center Report* 50 (3): 28–32. https://doi.org/10.1002/hast.1128

Hick, John L., Dan Hanfling, Matthew Wynia, and Eric Toner. 2021. "Crisis Standards of Care and COVID-19: What Did We Learn? How Do We Ensure Equity? What Should We Do?" *National Academy of Medicine*, August 30, 2021. https://doi.org/10.31478/202108e

Hu, J., A. J. H. Kind, and D. Nerenz. 2018. "Area Deprivation Index Predicts Readmission Risk at an Urban Teaching Hospital." *American Journal of Medical Quality* 33 (5): 493–501. https://doi.org/10.1177/1062860617753063

Iezzoni, L. I. 2011. "Eliminating health and health care disparities among the growing population of people with disabilities." *Health Affairs* 30 (10): 1947–1954. https://doi.org/10.1377/hlthaff.2011.0613

Iezzoni, L. I., S. R. Rao, J. Ressalam, D. Bolcic-Jankovic, N. D. Agaronnik, K. Donelan, T. Lagu, and E. G. Campbell. 2021. "Physicians' Perceptions of People with Disability and Their Health Care." *Health Affairs* 40 (2): 297–306. https://doi.org/10.1377/hlthaff.2020.01452

Institute of Medicine. 2010. *Summary of Guidance for Establishing Crisis Standards of Care for Use in Disaster Situations: A Letter Report, appendix B.* Washington, DC: National Academies Press.

Jones, C. P. 2000. "Levels of Racism: A Theoretic Framework and a Gardener's Tale." *American Journal of Public Health* 90 (8): 1212–1215. https://doi.org/10.2105/ajph.90.8.1212

Krahn, G. L.; Walker, D. K.; and Correa-De-Araujo, R. 2015. "Persons with Disabilities as an Unrecognized Health Disparity Population." *American Journal of Public Health* 105: S198–S206. https://doi.org/10.2105/AJPH.2014.302182

Landes, S. D., J. M. Finan, and M. A. Turk. 2022. "COVID-19 Mortality Burden and Comorbidity Patterns among Decedents with and without Intellectual and Developmental Disability in the US." *Disability and Health Journal* 15 (4): 101376. https://doi.org/10.1016/j.dhjo.2022.101376

Laventhal, N., R. Basak, M. L. Dell, D. Diekema, N. Elster, G. Geis, M. Mercurio, D. Opel, D. Shalowitz, M. Statter, and R. Macauley. 2020. "The Ethics of Creating a Resource Allocation Strategy During the COVID-19 Pandemic." *Pediatrics* 146 (1). https://doi.org/10.1542/peds.2020-1243

Lewis, Talila A. 2023. "Ableism Enables All Forms of Inequity and Hampers All Liberation Efforts." Interview by George Yancy. *Truthout*, January 3, 2023. https://truthout.org/articles/ableism-enables-all-forms-of-inequity-and-hampers-all-liberation-efforts/

Maves, R. C., J. Downar, J. R. Dichter, J. L. Hick, A. Devereaux, J. A. Geiling, N. Kissoon, N. Hupert, A. S. Niven, M. A. King, L. L. Rubinson, D. Hanfling, J. G. Hodge, Jr., M. F. Marshall, K. Fischkoff, L. E. Evans, M. R. Tonelli, R. S. Wax, G. Seda, J. S. Parrish, R. D. Truog, C. L. Sprung, M. D. Christian. 2020. "Triage of Scarce Critical Care Resources in COVID-19 An Implementation Guide for Regional Allocation: An Expert Panel Report of the Task Force for Mass Critical Care and the American College of Chest Physicians." *Chest* 158 (1): 212–225. https://doi.org/10.1016/j.chest.2020.03.063

Mello, M. M., G. Persad, and D. B. White. 2020. "Respecting Disability Rights - Toward Improved Crisis Standards of Care." *The New England Journal of Medicine* 383 (5): e26. https://doi.org/10.1056/NEJMp2011997

Miller, W. D., X. Han, M. E. Peek, D. Charan Ashana, and W. F. Parker. 2021. "Accuracy of the Sequential Organ Failure Assessment Score for In-Hospital Mortality by Race and Relevance to Crisis Standards of Care." *JAMA Network Open* 4 (6): e2113891. https://doi.org/10.1001/jamanetworkopen.2021.13891

National Academy of Medicine. 2020. "National Organizations Call for Action to Implement Crisis Standards of Care During COVID-19 Surge." *National Academy of Medicine*, December 18, 2020. https://nam.edu/national-organizations-call-for-action-to-implement-crisis-standards-of-care-during-covid-19-surge/

National Academies of Sciences, Engineering, and Medicine. 2020. *Framework for Equitable Allocation of COVID-19 Vaccine*. Edited by Helene Gayle, William Foege, Lisa Brown and Benjamin Kahn. Washington, DC: The National Academies Press.

National Academies of Sciences, Engineering and Medicine. 2020. *Rapid Expert Consultation on Crisis Standards of Care for the COVID-19 Pandemic (March 28, 2020)*. Washington, DC: The National Academies Press.

Ne'eman, A., M. A. Stein, Z. D. Berger, and D. Dorfman. 2021. "The Treatment of Disability under Crisis Standards of Care: An Empirical and Normative Analysis of Change over Time during COVID-19." *Journal of Health Politics, Policy, and Law* 46 (5): 831–860. https://doi.org/10.1215/03616878-9156005

Office for Civil Rights Actions. 2020. *Civil Rights, HIPSS, and the Coronavirus Disease 2019 (COVID-19)*. October 2, 2020. https://www.hhs.gov/sites/default/files/ocr-bulletin-3-28-20.pdf

Peña-Guzman, D. M., and J. M. Reynolds. 2019. "The Harm of Ableism: Medical Error and Epistemic Injustice." *Kennedy Institute Ethics Journal* 29 (3): 205–242. https://doi.org/10.1353/ken.2019.0023

Persad, G. 2021. "Against Exclusive Survivalism: Preventing Lost Life and Protecting the Disadvantaged in Resource Allocation." *Hastings Center Report* 51 (5): 47–51. https://doi.org/10.1002/hast.1286

Persad, G., A. Wertheimer, and E. J. Emanuel. 2009. "Principles for allocation of scarce medical interventions." *Lancet* 373 (9661): 423–431. https://doi.org/10.1016/S0140-6736(09).60137-9

Prusak, B., M. Gaurke, K. Y. Jeong, E. Scire, and D. P. Sulmasy. 2021. "ICU Care in a Pandemic." *Hastings Center Report* 51 (6): 58. https://doi.org/10.1002/hast.1309

Rajczi, A., J. Daar, A. Kheriaty, and C. Dastur. 2021. "The University of California Crisis Standards of Care: Public Reasoning for Socially Responsible Medicine." *Hastings Center Report* 51 (5): 30–41. https://doi.org/10.1002/hast.1284

Raschke, R. A., S. Agarwal, P. Rangan, C. W. Heise, and S. C. Curry. 2021. "Discriminant Accuracy of the SOFA Score for Determining the Probable Mortality of Patients With COVID-19 Pneumonia Requiring Mechanical Ventilation." *JAMA* 325 (14): 1469–1470. https://doi.org/10.1001/jama.2021.1545

Reynolds, J. M. 2018. "Three Things Clinicians Should Know About Disability." *AMA Journal of Ethics* 20 (12): E1181–1187. https://doi.org/10.1001/amajethics.2018.1181

Reynolds, J. M., L. Guidry-Grimes, and K. Savin. 2021. "Against Personal Ventilator Reallocation." *Cambridge Quarterly of Healthcare Ethics* 30 (2): 272–284. https://doi.org/10.1017/S0963180120000833

Rollston, R., and S. Galea. 2020. "COVID-19 and the Social Determinants of Health." *Cambridge Quarterly of Healthcare Ethics* 34 (6): 687–689. https://doi.org/10.1177/0890117120930536b

Sabatello, M., T. B. Burke, K. E. McDonald, and P. S. Appelbaum. 2020. "Disability, Ethics, and Health Care in the COVID-19 Pandemic." *American Journal of Public Health* 110 (10): 1523–1527. https://doi.org/10.2105/AJPH.2020.305837

Sanchez-Pinto, L. N., W. F. Parker, A. Mayampurath, S. Derrington, and K. N. Michelson. 2021. "Evaluation of Organ Dysfunction Scores for Allocation of Scarce Resources in Critically Ill Children and Adults During a Healthcare Crisis." *Critical Care Medicine* 49 (2): 271–281. https://doi.org/10.1097/CCM.0000000000004774

Savin, K. and Guidry-Grimes, L. 2020. "Confronting Disability Discrimination During the Pandemic." *The Hastings Center*, April 2, 2020. https://thehastingscenter.org/confronting-disability-discrimination-during-the-pandemic/

Scheunemann, L. P., and D. B. White. 2011. "The Ethics and Reality of Rationing in Medicine." *Chest* 140 (6): 1625–1632. https://doi.org/10.1378/chest.11-0622

Schmidt, H., D. E. Roberts, and N. D. Eneanya. 2022. "Rationing, Racism and Justice: Advancing the Debate Around 'colourblind' COVID-19 Ventilator Allocation." *Journal of Medical Ethics* 48 (2): 126–130. https://doi.org/10.1136/medethics-2020-106856. https://www.ncbi.nlm.nih.gov/pubmed/33408091

Schmidt, H., Gostin, L. O., and Williams, M. A. 2020. "Is It Lawful and Ethical to Prioritize Racial Minorities for COVID-19 Vaccines?" *JAMA* 324 (20): 2023–2024.

Schmidt, H., Shaikh, S. J., Sadecki, E., and Buttenheim, A. et al. 2022. "Public Attitudes About Equitable COVID-19 Vaccine Allocation: A Randomised Experiment of Race-based versus Novel Place-based Frames." *Journal of Medical Ethics* 48 (12): 993–999.

National Academy of Science. 2012. *Crisis Standards of Care: A Systems Framework for Catastrophic Disaster Response: Volume 1: Introduction and CSC Framework*. Washington, DC: National Academies Press.

Scully, J. L. 2020. "Disability, Disablism, and COVID-19 Pandemic Triage." *Journal of Bioethical Inquiry* 17 (4): 601–605. https://doi.org/10.1007/s11673-020-10005-y

Office for Civil Rights. 2022. "FAQs for Healthcare Providers during the COVID-19 Public Health Emergency: Federal Civil Rights Protections for Individuals with Disabilities under Section 504 and Section 1557." *U.S. Department of Health and Human Services*, February 4, 2022. https://www.hhs.gov/civil-rights/for-providers/civil-rights-covid19/disabilty-faqs/index.html

Smith, Leah. 2023. "#Ableism." *Center for Disability Rights*. cdrnys.org/blog/uncategorized/ableism

Solomon, M. Z., M. K. Wynia, and L. O. Gostin. 2020. "COVID-19 Crisis Triage - Optimizing Health Outcomes and Disability Rights." *The New England Journal of Medicine* 383 (5): e27. https://doi.org/10.1056/NEJMp2008300

Tai, D. B. G., A. Shah, C. A. Doubeni, I. G. Sia, and M. L. Wieland. 2021. "The Disproportionate Impact of COVID-19 on Racial and Ethnic Minorities in the United States." *Clinical Infectious Diseases* 72 (4): 703–706. https://doi.org/10.1093/cid/ciaa815

Tolchin, B., C. Oladele, D. Galusha, N. Kashyap, M. Showstark, J. Bonito, M. C. Salazar, J. L. Herbst, S. Martino, N. Kim, K. A. Nash, M. J. Nguemeni Tiako, S. Roy, R. Vergara Greeno, and K. Jubanyik. 2021. "Racial Disparities in the SOFA Score among Patients Hospitalized with COVID-19." *PLoS One* 16 (9): e0257608. https://doi.org/10.1371/journal.pone.0257608

Turk, M. A., S. D. Landes, M. K. Formica, and K. D. Goss. 2020. "Intellectual and Developmental Disability and COVID-19 Case-Fatality Trends: TriNetX Analysis." *Disability and Health Journal* 13 (3): 100942. https://doi.org/10.1016/j.dhjo.2020.100942

University of California Critical Care Bioethics Working Group. June 17, 2020. *Allocation of Scarce Critical Resources under Crisis Standards of Care*. University of California (California). https://www.ucop.edu/uc-health/reports-resources/uc-critical-care-bioethics-working-group-report-rev-6-17-20.pdf

White, D. B.; Katz, M. H.; Luce, J. M.; and Lo, B. 2009. "Who Should Receive Life Support During a Public Health Emergency? Using Ethical Principles to Improve Allocation Decisions." *Annals of Internal Medicine* 150 (2): 132–138.

White D. B. and Lo, B. 2020. "A Framework for Rationing Ventilators and Critical Care Beds During the COVID-19 Pandemic." *JAMA* 323 (18): 1773–1774.

White, D. B., and B. Lo. 2021. "Mitigating Inequities and Saving Lives with ICU Triage during the COVID-19 Pandemic." *American Journal of Respiratory and Critical Care Medicine* 203 (3): 287–295. https://doi.org/10.1164/rccm.202010-3809CP

White, D., and B. Lo. 2022. "Promoting Equity with a Multi-principle Framework to Allocate Scarce ICU Resources." *Journal of Medical Ethics* 48 (2): 133–135. https://doi.org/10.1136/medethics-2021-107456

Yancy, C. W. 2020. "COVID-19 and African Americans." *JAMA* 323 (19): 1891–1892. https://doi.org/10.1001/jama.2020.6548

3

TRAGIC CHOICES

Disability, Triage, and Equity Amidst a Global Pandemic

Joseph A. Stramondo

In the Spring of 2020, bioethicists and physicians scrambling to develop triage protocols for the COVID-19 crisis might have been surprised that counsel from Self Advocates in Leadership (SAIL), Disability Rights Washington (DRW), and The Arc of the United States (The Arc) filed a complaint with the U.S. Department of Health and Human Services (HHS) Office for Civil Rights (OCR) over their concerns regarding disability discrimination in some of these protocols (Carlson et al. 2020).[1] Perhaps it would have been easy to dismiss such concerns as mere naivete that failed to recognize the inevitability of the hard choices coming down the pike in the United States. After all, "none of the above" is not one of the choices available for the Trolley Problem. Such a dismissal would have been a serious mistake. More specifically, those who developed these protocols would have done well to pay attention to the critiques of bioethical reasoning that were made both by disability activists at the beginning of the pandemic (Kukla 2020) and by disability studies scholars who have consistently and substantively engaged with these issues for decades (Cureton and Wasserman 2020).

Several clinical bioethicists asked me what sorts of triage criteria *would* satisfy the disability critiques of these protocols (Disability Rights Education and Defense Fund 2020). As with most questions in bioethics, there is no easy answer. Of course, just because there may not be a perfect, non-discriminatory set of rationing criteria, that does not mean there are not better or worse ways of doing triage. Let me review some of the triage criteria that I will argue are on the "worse" side of ledger.

First, consider any criterion that deprioritizes people with specific disabilities as a group. A *New York Times* op-ed by Ari Ne'eman (2020) brought our attention to these kinds of protocols in the context of the COVID-19 pandemic, including Alabama's protocol denying ventilators to folks with "severe or profound" intellectual disabilities under the state's initial Emergency Operations Plan (Alabama Department of Public Health 2010) and Tennessee's original protocol denying treatment to those with spinal muscular atrophy who require help with activities of daily living (Tennessee Altered Standards of Care Workgroup 2016).

I would argue that this sort of criterion is clearly grounded in a deeply biased quality-of-life judgment. Unlike supporting a patient's right to request the withdrawal of life-sustaining care, or even requesting assistance in dying, denying patients care on the basis of a non-terminal

DOI: 10.4324/9781003502623-5

disability is not justified via the principle of respect for a patient's autonomy and self-assessment regarding their own quality of life. Rather, the reason why such a person would be denied life-saving care via triage is because a third-party judge, like a physician or policy maker, does not believe that their life has enough quality to be worth saving in comparison with that of non-disabled others. A person's self-assessment of their own well-being is deemed irrelevant in the context of triage, and thus, I would argue, any third-party assessment of a person's well-being should also be deemed irrelevant.

Of course, there is a significant body of empirical evidence showing that there is a substantial gap between how a disabled person's quality of life is assessed by the disabled person themself rather than by people that have never experienced their disability. Some prominent bioethicists even refer to this as the "disability paradox." I would maintain that it is not paradoxical for disabled people to value their own lives more than non-disabled people do, making judgments based on stereotype and stigma (Amundson 2010). To conceptualize this gap in assessment and valuation as paradoxical is to wrongly assume that disability inevitably diminishes well-being. This assumption is a central tenant of what Amundson calls the "ideology" of ableism because it grounds the notion that the disadvantages of disability are intrinsic and inevitable, rather than socially constructed, and thus, ameliorable via social interventions, like civil rights laws (Amundson 2005).

Some of the triage protocols developed early in the COVID-19 pandemic avoided singling out particular disabilities that are presumed to make life barely worth living, but these protocols that deployed more sweeping generalizations were still as problematic. For example, the University of Washington Medical Center's "Material Resource Allocation Principles and Guidelines," which form the basis of the HHS OCR complaint, avoided this rationale that focused on the categorical exclusion of people with specific disabilities. However, it used the concept of "health," instead, as a proxy for quality of life (University of Washington Medical Center 2020). This might be even more morally troubling because it was not as obviously prejudicial to the average observer.

In my view, this reliance on an allegedly objective and unbiased concept of health was the biggest flaw in the University of Washington's original guidelines. This protocol explicitly committed itself to utilitarian principles as the basis of triage, and then stated that the

> greatest good, in a protracted clinical situation such as the COVID-19 outbreak, is generally considered maximizing survival of patients with COVID-19…Overall survival may be further qualified as healthy, long-term survival, recognizing that this represents weighting the survival of young otherwise healthy patients more heavily than that of older, chronically debilitated patients.
>
> *(University of Washington Medical Center 2020)*

This should be read as an attempt to smuggle in a quality-of-life criterion for triage because health is meant to equate to well-being in this context.

One might think that this reading is mistaken and that health was not actually a proxy for quality of life in this protocol. Perhaps there are legitimate reasons why health should be considered during triage, such as the intuition that a "healthy" person is more likely to survive than someone who is "chronically debilitated." Indeed, we don't want to waste scarce resources on people who will not survive, even with treatment. However, this clearly is not what this original University of Washington protocol called for. Likelihood of survival and general health come apart conceptually, and in fact, they were parsed in this protocol. Upon a close reading it was adding health as a criterion on top of the criterion concerning likelihood of survival. In other words, the way this protocol was worded did not aim to maximize the survival of everyone, but rather, to maximize the survival of people who will be "healthy" (i.e. non-disabled) after receiving treatment.

It may just be the case that this initial University of Washington protocol was recommending that people with a bad prognosis for overall survival, separate from their experience with COVID-19, be deprioritized. Maybe all that was being recommended was that folks with, say, pancreatic cancer should not receive aggressive treatment because, even if they have as good a likelihood as anyone else of surviving the virus, they are not likely to survive much longer after that. However, health and disease are notoriously broad, vague concepts in medicine (Kukla 2014). Thus, we must ask if these guidelines from University of Washington would have recommended withholding critical care from someone who is "chronically debilitated" because, for instance, they are blind or deaf or they have achondroplasia or a spinal cord injury. Without further specification (i.e. language about having a near-term terminal diagnosis), it seems that many things could disqualify someone from treatment because they will not be "healthy," even after they recover. To be sure, this was the aim of the protocol in that it assumed health equates to quality of life. Such an assumption would not just ignore the self-assessment of many disabled people but would also dismiss a rapidly growing scholarly literature arguing that it is simply false to believe that disabled people tend to be worse off (Barnes 2016; Campbell and Stramondo 2017).

In sum, I would argue that any triage protocol is unjustly discriminatory against disabled people insofar as it deprioritizes them due to a belief that their lives are of less value because they are of less quality. However, what about the triage strategy of assessing the likelihood that a patient will survive COVID-19, even with aggressive treatment? As already conceded, on the face of it, this seems safer from ableist bias than the previously examined quality-of-life criterion. After all, even someone who rejects utilitarian ethics out of hand would likely not advocate for patients to be provided with truly futile care that will not actually help them survive the virus and save their life.

Yet, judging the futility of treatment is a rather inexact science under the best of circumstances, and in the context of pandemic triage, what we are really talking about is not futility, but a scale of likelihood of survival. That is, especially given the lack of detailed, accurate knowledge about the variable effects of a new virus in the time of a pandemic, there will not be a bright, clearly discernable line between those for whom treatment is absolutely futile and those who are merely unlikely to survive. Further, there will be significant overlap between the population of patients that are unlikely to survive even with treatment and those that have disabilities, some of which will entail comorbid risk factors. However, this isn't itself an argument that such a likelihood-of-survival criterion is necessarily unfairly biased in the same way that a quality-of-life criterion seems to have ableist bias baked right into it.

If and when tragic choices need to be made, it seems that some disabilities are relevant insofar as they are associated with comorbidities that we are reasonably sure will reduce the likelihood that a patient will respond to treatment and survive. There is still a risk of ableist bias finding its way into the application of this sort of likelihood-of-survival criterion, but there are ways to reduce this risk. A deeper concern is whether we ought to also deprioritize, on the same grounds, disabled folks that may have as good a likelihood of surviving as anyone else but may require more treatment to get there. We can call this the level-of-resource-intensity criterion. Ultimately, the question is: Can we consistently justify excluding patients that are less likely to survive in order to conserve resources, and thus, save more lives, without also excluding patients who will use more than an average amount of resources to survive? I think we can.

Given that there is still so much to learn about COVID-19 and its variants, there are going to be as many questions as certainties when making judgments about how various comorbidities effect prognosis. Data have become more reliable over the course of the crisis, but these data seem to have significant limits due to the enormous variation between patients, even those sharing the same diagnosis. Consider the case highlighted in the press release announcing the legal action against the state of Washington:

> I am concerned that a doctor will see my diagnosis of cystic fibrosis in my chart and make lots of erroneous assumptions about me. Cystic fibrosis often comes with significant breathing difficulties and a life expectancy of 30 years…However, tests show that I have better breathing capacity than most people without cystic fibrosis…
>
> *(Katz 2020)*

I think the worry being expressed here is that, in its application, the likelihood-of-survival criterion will sometimes slip into ableist bias by relying on disability as a heuristic. As Jackie Leach Scully puts it in her discussion of using likelihood of survival as a triage criterion, since disabled people are stereotypically assumed to be ill, "individual differences mean global rules (of the "no one with cystic fibrosis to be placed on ventilation" kind) could easily be unjust" (Scully 2020). So, even if people with disability X that typically occurs with comorbidity Y are less likely to survive in general, we ought to do our best to ensure that actual person P with disability X truly has comorbidity Y before denying treatment. Otherwise, there is a good chance that the denial is being motivated by stereotype rather than evidence. This is the sort of scenario the HHS Office of Civil Rights' recent bulletin is trying to account for when it states that "whether an individual is a candidate for treatment should be based on an individualized assessment of the patient based on the best available objective medical evidence" (2020).

Feminist bioethicist Alison Reiheld has argued that some kind of feedback loop would be the best way to account for these biases by motivating more nuanced triage decisions by conducting high level oversite that looks for patterns of bias.[2] Such a procedural safeguard would involve hospitals conducting reviews of triage decisions against treating someone who would have been a candidate for treatment under ordinary circumstances. This is not to say that such decisions are inherently discriminatory. After all, these are not ordinary circumstances. However, this broad oversite could serve as a trigger for closer examination of certain complex cases, thus motivating triage committees to look more closely at such cases from the get-go. In this way, watching for ableist bias in the misapplication of the likelihood-of-survival criterion may decrease assessment errors in which a person is unfairly assumed, contrary to evidence, to have a lower likelihood of survival because of a disability.

The motivation behind denying resources to people that are less likely to survive is to conserve those resources, which can then be used to save others who are more likely to survive, in an attempt to maximize the number of lives saved. If we endorse this kind of thinking, are we then committed to then *withholding* resources from those who have a good chance of survival, but only by using more resources? After all, this too would increase the number of people who survive by spreading the total amount of life-saving resources across a greater number of criti-cally ill patients. Yet, I actually think we can consistently accept the likelihood-of-survival criterion while rejecting this other level-of-resource-intensity criterion, even if both aim at maximizing the number of lives saved.

According to the first likelihood-of-survival criterion, patients that fall below a certain threshold of likelihood that they will survive may be turned away because these scarce resources may be *wasted*. This is the scenario in which the ICU bed is filled, the ventilator is in use, and yet the patient dies. According to the second level-of-resource-intensity criterion, even though it may take more resources to get the job done, those resources aren't wasted because they save someone's life. This may be *inefficient* but is surely not wasteful. Inefficiency implies that a resource was not used to achieve its maximum benefit. Waste implies that a resource was not used to achieve any benefit.

It would be a serious moral error to conflate these two scenarios. Harking back all the way to the American eugenics movement, there is a long, grim history of confusing inefficiency with wastefulness when it comes to the fair treatment of disabled people. One could even con-ceptualize the entire disability rights movement as an attempt to draw this distinction. It may reduce efficiency to bring disabled people into the mainstream of education, employment, and so on, but that does not mean that the resources used to do this are wasted. I see no reason why we can't draw this same distinction when it comes to triage. By ignoring the level-of-resource-intensity criterion, it is true that fewer lives may be saved, but perhaps it would guar-antee greater fairness when it comes to individuals' chances to access care that they would benefit from (Ballantyne 2020). This sort of fairness would not be a waste.

Thankfully, at the time at which I am drafting this essay in the summer of 2021, most regions and hospitals have been able to avoid activating crisis standards of care in response to the COVID-19 pandemic. What's better is that, due to legal and political pressure, many of the most discriminatory of these protocols have been revised over the course of the crisis, including the most problematic of those referenced above (Ne'eman et al. 2021).

Paradoxically, maybe most communities avoided having to make these tragic choices by *not* focusing their attention and effort on preparing for them. Indeed, by narrowly focusing on triage protocols and by deeming them the most morally salient problem that we have faced during this unprecedented era, perhaps bioethics as a field has not been advancing the most important conversation. Towards the beginning of the pandemic, Shelley Tremain, a feminist philosopher of disability, argued that bioethicists should shift the focus of the conversation because targeting these protocols as the primary object of our analysis, at least indirectly, sanctioned the idea that these hard choices were inevitabilities. Rather than carefully parsing how to fairly deny treatment to some patients in order to maximize the number of lives saved, Tremain maintains that we, as professional bioethicists, should have been putting our energy behind efforts to reduce the need to make such choices at all (Tremain 2020). Arguably, Tremain was correct that it was, ultimately, the efforts to slow the spread of the disease and increase our structural capacity to treat it that minimized the number of lives lost.

As we made great efforts to slow the spread of the virus by eliminating or radically altering all sorts of features of our daily lives, it became more and more obvious that the presumed need for triage was driven by economic, political, and personal choices, not an inevitable march of events (Porter and Tankersley 2020). Without a vaccine or effective treatment, the only means available for reducing the death toll were masking, social distancing, sheltering in place, and so on. These practices were quickly politicized, largely because of how they would impact people financially in the context of late-stage capitalism. Adherence to these practices and eventually vaccination, or lack thereof, have been the most significant variables determining the extent of the crisis. In this context, Tremain suggested that bioethicists, as a field, ought to have been putting our work into prompting individual and structural efforts to keep infection rates down and triage protocols locked away.

What Tremain was suggesting was a powerful paradigm shift. If maximizing the number of people saved was the top priority of professional bioethics, we should have put ourselves and our considerable social capital to work in the service of slowing down the spread of the virus and building the capacity of the medical response. While we may not be engineers, nurses, physicians, or manufacturers who can work directly to make up for the shortfall in material and human resources available to those with the greatest need, Tremain argued there are some very specific ways that bioethicists could have worked to reduce the need for triage, which likely would have saved many more lives than perfecting a triage protocol.

First, we should have done more to collectively respond forcefully and persistently against politicians' constant flirtation with the idea that we should prematurely return to life as usual in the name of economics (Liptak and Collins 2020). Flattening the curve of the infection rate was our only effective means of reducing the unmet need for resources. As the virus has continued to spread via emerging variants and people have continued to die, arguments that prioritize the financial well-being of the politically powerful over the very lives of the politically vulnerable are nothing short of eugenic and bioethicists are positioned to point that out. It is clear that those impacted most by the virus, both in terms of health and finances, are poor, non-white, and disabled people, and thus, the U.S. is in a position where the most effective response would be a significant expansion of the social safety net, but this is often seen as a non-starter within basic liberal, capitalist social structures. That is, the kind of robust social support that would allow people to shelter in place rather than exposing themselves to the virus in order to meet their basic economic needs has been forcefully resisted by corporate interests because of the implications for redistributing wealth. Thus, neither of the two major political parties sees this as a viable political move. Fundamentally, though, this is a moral issue. Specifically, it is a question of public health ethics that bioethicists should have been willing to address. Put most starkly, it is deeply immoral to trade the lives of the most vulnerable for shareholder dividends and professional bioethicists need to say so.

Ultimately, professional bioethicists concerned with matters of justice are well positioned to make the case that there is a moral imperative to "flatten the curve" in order to save lives and to prioritize the public good over the limited interests of the economically and politically powerful. Zeke Emanuel's very good article in *The New York Times*, "Fourteen Days. That's the Most Time We Have to Defeat Coronavirus" (2020), is an example of how a bioethicist can show leadership on this issue. Of course, not all of us have the megaphone of an Emanuel brother. Even still, in my view, it is important that the public facing work bioethicists have been producing during the pandemic balances a discussion of triage protocol with a discussion of how the U.S. can take steps to avoid the nightmare scenario of triage by creating the public infrastructure to support the most socially and politically vulnerable rather than focusing mostly on how to ration healthcare resources amongst this same population. Part of this argument should be an explicit acknowledgement that a failure to do so is driven by a eugenic ideology.

Crucially, this approach to saving lives in the context of a pandemic is consistent with the political paradigm of disability justice, as I understand it. A disability justice paradigm, as opposed to the politics of disability rights as they have been typically practiced, prioritizes the epistemic position and the well-being of multiply marginalized disabled people. This means that a disability justice approach is explicitly intersectional, focusing on the experiences of disabled people who are also queer, poor, racialized, and so on. It is also explicitly critical and challenges the ways in which the disability rights movement has typically approached activism by seeking the inclusion of those disabled people with the most social power – cishet middle aged middle class white men – into the existing liberal, capitalist social structure, rather than trying to dismantle that structure (Piepzna-Samarasinha 2018). Focusing on reducing infection rates via a dramatic expansion of the social safety net, rather than focusing on triage protocols, clearly aligns with this intersectional, critical approach to disability politics. Further, offering explicitly anti-eugenic justification for these interventions is also a way of invoking an intersectional lens, since eugenic ideology is as much about race, class, gender, and sexuality as it is about disability. In this way, the response to the pandemic Tremain suggested interventions at least implicitly prioritized the epistemic position and the well-being of Queer, poor, BIPOC disabled people in the way that disability justice calls for.

It is also worth noting that the work of justifying these sorts of interventions is squarely in the purview of bioethics. Tremain has herself been deeply critical of the field of bioethics (Tremain 2017), but the interventions she suggested for preventing death during the earliest days of the COVID-19 pandemic can be easily justified in terms that appeal to even the most mainstream camps in the field. For example, protecting people at the margins of society by expanding the social safety net in times of public health crisis can be justified by appealing to mainstream interpretations of three of the four major bioethical principles defended by Beauchamp and Childress in their seminal text: justice, beneficence, and nonmaleficence (Beauchamp and Childress 2019). To be sure, there is no question that bioethics should be making these kinds of arguments with force and frequency.

While I don't fault clinical ethicists for making a good faith effort to work on thoughtful triage protocols that try to take account of ableist bias, even if it is impossible to eliminate it altogether, it would be a serious mistake for professional bioethics as a whole to exclusively focus on triage protocols in their public work, rather than calling for an end to the kinds of large scale, systemic injustices that have hindered the country's ability to minimize the amount that triage has even been necessary.

Acknowledgments

I would like to thank the following individuals and groups for providing fertile conversation about the questions I address in this paper and feedback on earlier drafts that greatly improved its quality: Lori Bruce, Craig Klugman, David Wasserman, Ari Ne'eman, Leah Smith, Stephen M. Campbell, Marina Tsaplina, David Carlson, Alice Wong, Jess Whatcott, Catherine Clune-Taylor, Shelley Tremain, Dominic Sisti, Hanna Shaul Bar Nissim, Laura Guidry-Grimes, Katie Savin, Joel Michael Reynolds, Teresa Blankmeyer Burke, Angela Ballantyne, Eva Feder Kittay, Devan Stahl, Jackie Leach Scully, Rosemarie Garland-Thomson, Anita Tarzian, Doron Dorfman, Joseph J. Fins, the Nuland Summer Institute in Bioethics at Yale University, the Radcliffe Institute for Advanced Study at Harvard University, the American Medical Association's Ethics Talk Podcast, the University of Washington Student Disability Commission, and the Disability Visibility Podcast, and the copy-editors at the Journal of Philosophy of Disability.

Notes

1 This chapter is reprinted from Joseph A. Stramondo, "Tragic Choices: Disability, Triage, and Equity Amidst a Global Pandemic," *Journal of Philosophy of Disability* 1: 201–210, 2021. https://doi.org/10.5840/jpd20219206.
2 Personal Correspondence March 2020.

Work Cited

Alabama Department of Public Health. 2010. *Annex to ESF 8 of the State of Alabama Emergency Operations Plan Criteria for Mechanical Ventilator Triage Following Proclamation of Mass-Casualty Respiratory Emergency.* April 9, 2010. http://www.adph.org/CEP/assets/VENTTRIAGE.pdf (Accessed March 29, 2020. This source has since been removed from the Alabama Public Health website and is no longer available online.)

Amundson, Ronald. 2005. "Disability, Ideology, and Quality of Life: A Bias in Biomedical Ethics." In *Quality of Life and Human Difference: Genetic Testing, Health Care, and Disability*, eds. David Wasserman, Jerome Bickenbach, and Robert Wachbroit, 101–124. New York: Cambridge University Press. https://doi.org/10.1017/cbo9780511614590.005

Amundson, Ronald. 2010. "Quality of Life, Disability, ad Hedonic Psychology." *Journal for the Theory of Social Behaviour* 40 (4): 374–392. https://doi.org/10.1111/j.1468-5914.2010.00437.x

Ballantyne, Angela. 2020. "ICU Triage: How many lives or whose lives?" *Blog: Journal of Medical Ethics*, April 7, 2020. https://blogs.bmj.com/medical-ethics/2020/04/07/icu-triage-how-many-lives-or-whose-lives/

Barnes, Elizabeth. 2016. *The Minority Body: A Theory of Disability*. Oxford: Oxford University Press. https://doi.org/10.1093/acprof:oso/9780198732587.001.0001

Beauchamp, Tom L. and James F. Childress. 2019. *Principles of Biomedical Ethics*, 8th ed. Oxford University Press.

Campbell, Stephen, and Joseph Stramondo. 2017. "The Complicated Relationship of Disability and WellBeing" *The Kennedy Institute for Ethics Journal* 27 (2): 151–184. https://doi.org/10.1353/ken.2017.0014

Carlson, David, Jennifer Mathis, Samantha Crane, Shira Wakschlag, Cathy Costanzo, and Samuel Bagenstos. 2020. "Complaint of Disability Rights Washington, Self-Advocates in Leadership, The Arc of the United States, and Ivanova Smith Against the Washington State Department of Health (WA DOH), the Northwest Healthcare Response Network (NHRN) and the University of Washington Medical Center (UWMC)." *The Arc of the United States.* http://thearc.org/wp-content/uploads/2020/03/OCR-Complaint_3-23-20.pdf

Cureton, Adam, and David Wasserman, eds. 2020. *The Oxford Handbook of Philosophy and Disability.* Oxford University Press. https://doi.org/10.1093/oxfordhb/9780190622879.001.0001

Disability Rights Education and Defense Fund. 2020. "Preventing Discrimination in the Treatment of COVID19 Patients: The Illegality of Medical Rationing on the Basis of Disability." *DREDF.org.* https://dredf.org/wp-content/uploads/2020/03/DREDF-Policy-Statement-on-COVID-19-and-Medical-Rationing-3-25-2020.pdf

Emanuel, Ezekiel. 2020. "Fourteen Days. That's the Most Time We Have to Defeat Coronavirus." *The New York Times*, March 23, 2020. https://www.nytimes.com/2020/03/23/opinion/contributors/us-coronavirus-response.html

U.S. Office of Civil Rights. 2020. *Civil Rights, HIPAA, and the Coronavirus Disease 2019*. Washington, DC: Department of Health and Human Services. https://www.hhs.gov/sites/default/files/ocr-bulletin-3-28-20.pdf

Katz, Pam. 2020. "Disability Discrimination Complaint Filed Over COVID19 Treatment Rationing Plan in Washington State." *The Arc of the United States*, March 23, 2020. https://thearc.org/disability-discrimination-complaint-filed-over-covid-19-treatment-rationing-plan-in-washington-state/

Kukla, Elliot. 2020. "My Life Is More Disposable During This Pandemic: The ableism and ageism being unleashed is its own sort of pestilence." *The New York Times*, March 19, 2020. https://www.nytimes.com/2020/03/19/opinion/coronavirus-disabled-health-care.html

Kukla, Rebecca. 2014. "Medicalization, "Normal Function," and the Definition of Health." In *The Routledge Companion to Bioethics*, eds. John D. Arras, Elizabeth Fenton, and Rebecca Kukla, 515–530. New York: Routledge. https://doi.org/10.4324/9780203804971

Liptak, Kevin, and Kaitlan Collins. 2020. "Trump Spends Easter Weekend Pondering the 'Biggest Decision' of his Presidency." *CNN*, April 11, 2020. https://www.cnn.com/2020/04/11/politics/donald-trump-coronavirus-economy-testing/index.html

Ne'eman, Ari. 2020. "I Will Not Apologize for My Needs: Even in crisis, doctors should not abandon the principle of nondiscrimination." *The New York Times*, March 23, 2020. https://www.nytimes.com/2020/03/23/opinion/coronavirus-ventilators-triage-disability.html

Ne'eman, Ari, Michael Ashley Stein, Zackary D. Berger, and Doron Dorfman. 2021. "The Treatment of Disability Under Crisis Standards of Care: An Empirical and Normative Analysis of Change Over Time During COVID-19." *Journal of Health Politics, Policy and Law* 46 (5): 831–860. https://doi.org/10.1215/03616878-9156005

Piepzna-Samarasinha, Leah Lakshmi. 2018. *Care Work: Dreaming Disability Justice*. Arsenal Pulp Press.

Porter, Eduardo, and Jim Tankersley. 2020. "Shutdown Spotlights Economic Cost of Saving Lives: President Trump and others have asked if halting normal life and commerce to fight the coronavirus is worth the cost. Here's how economists figure it." *The New York Times*, April 13, 2020. https://www.nytimes.com/2020/03/24/business/economy/coronavirus-economy.html

Scully, Jackie Leach. 2020. "Disablism in a Time of Pandemic: Some Things Don't Change." *International Journal of Feminist Approaches to Bioethics Blog*, April 1, 2020. https://www.ijfab.org/blog/2020/04/disablism-in-a-time-of-pandemic-some-things-dont-change/

Tennessee Altered Standards of Care Workgroup. 2016. "Guidance for the Ethical Allocation of Scarce Resources during a Community-Wide Public Health Emergency as Declared by the Governor of Tennessee." Tennessee Department of Health. Version 1.6 (July 2016, revised 2020). https://www.tn.gov/content/dam/tn/health/documents/cedep/ep/Guidance_for_the_Ethical_Allocation_of_Scarce_Resources.pdf

Tremain, Shelley. 2020. "COVID-19, Face Shields, and 3-D Printers." *Biopolitical Philosophy*, March 23, 2020. https://biopoliticalphilosophy.com/2020/03/23/covid-19-face-shields-and-3d-printers/

Tremain, Shelley. 2017. *Foucault and Feminist Philosophy of Disability*. University of Michigan Press.

University of Washington Medical Center. 2020. "Material Resource Allocation: Principles and Guidelines: COVID-19 Outbreak." *University of Washington Medicine: COVID-19*. https://covid19.uwmedicine.org/Screening%20and%20Testing%20Algorithms/Other%20Inpatient%20Clinical%20Guidance/Clinical%20Care%20in%20ICU/Material%20Resource%20Allocation.COVID19.docx. (This source has since been removed from the UW Medicine website and is no longer available online.)

PART II
Multiply Marginalized

4

"WE ARE A COMPROMISE"

A Social Security Model of Disability During COVID-19

Katie Savin

Introduction

When COVID-19 was declared a pandemic in March 2020, I was a PhD student recently booted off Social Security Disability Insurance (SSDI) due to the income I received from academic fellowships and grants. I was becoming familiar with the academic literature in the field of Social Security disability policy and finding that it seemed to be relatively uninformed by lived experience. The knowledge I had gained from my experience receiving Social Security disability benefits and from my interactions with fellow beneficiaries was not reflected in the research but felt relevant to the questions being posed by researchers. I saw my position as a person in transition from SSDI beneficiary to academic as ideally suited to systematize this hard-won knowledge concerning how disabled people survive on Social Security disability benefits (both the public assistance program, Supplemental Security Income, or SSI and the social insurance program, Social Security Disability Insurance). I knew my disabled community's struggles to make ends meet and to navigate a complex policy administration environment resulted in near-constant crisis. Their financial, social, and health-related conditions interacted to create conditions of extreme precarity. While the financial and social oppression of disabled life in the United States breeds a disabled ingenuity born out of the struggle for survival, I hoped translating these experiences into the language of policymaking might amplify the voices of disabled people in service of a more just world.

Though I did not set out to explore the impact of emergency conditions beyond the daily emergencies faced in poverty—such as the efforts to access enough food and medicine to survive each day—the COVID-19 pandemic created a natural experiment of managing quotidian crisis in emergency pandemic conditions. When the lockdowns were first implemented in California in 2020, I still had about two thirds of my dissertation interviews left to conduct. As a high-risk disabled researcher interviewing vulnerable, disabled adults, I quickly pivoted to phone and video conferences for my interviews. I did not change the focus of my interviews; however, I knew the impact of COVID-19 would become inextricable from my questions on daily survival and sense of self, and thus added a question to my interview guide

DOI: 10.4324/9781003502623-7

explicitly asking about participants' COVID-related experiences. This chapter will explore the impact of a global pandemic on the experience of managing life's daily emergencies as disabled adults living in poverty in California's Bay Area.

Background

Even prior to the COVID-19 pandemic, the 13 million adults in the United States under the age of 65 who received SSI and/or SSDI benefits as their primary source of income had to navigate a complex web of social welfare policies, interlocking benefit programs, and social stigma. SSI and SSDI programs provide monthly cash benefits to eligible beneficiaries. SSI benefit amounts are based on a federal standard maximum monthly amount which in 2019, at the time this study began, was $771 for an individual and $1,157 for a couple (Social Security Administration [SSA] 2020). Their benefit amounts leave over 40% of these individuals living in poverty (operationalized as about $12,800 per person per year according to the US federal poverty level, which many argue is far too low, particularly for high cost of living regions such as California's Bay Area where this study took place). The relationship between maximum monthly SSI and average monthly SSDI benefit levels and the Federal Poverty Level is depicted below. The fact that *SSA policy dictates poverty* for many disabled Americans cannot be over-emphasized, as the conditions of disability and poverty, while often erroneously conflated and treated as a natural fact, are *designed to be linked* through SSA policy (Goodley, Lawthom, and Runswick-Cole 2014) (Figure 4.1).

The experience of living on SSI and SSDI benefits goes beyond the receipt of a very low income. Beneficiaries must follow complex and outdated rules, such as SSI's limit of $2,000 in assets in order to maintain benefits, which has not been updated since the 1980s (Center on Budget and Policy Priorities 2022). To enforce this policy, SSI routinely surveils its beneficiaries' bank accounts, threatening to take away benefits from those who violate this policy. Hence, the SSA is an institution with significant power to shape the disability experience.

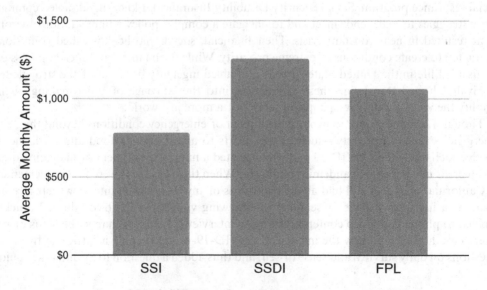

FIGURE 4.1   Comparison of SSI & SSDI Benefits to Federal Poverty Level (2020).

This power ranges from determining who is deemed disabled, setting income levels, providing income, and making rules disabled beneficiaries must follow in order to maintain their cash benefits, to encoding a widely accepted definition of disability as a status in contradistinction to participation in the labor market. By defining disability as an inability to work (due to medical reasons), the SSA creates a binary of labor market participation that precludes disabled beneficiaries from participating in it. Outside of the formal labor market, disabled beneficiaries must develop their own informal strategies to make ends meet. These strategies are often creative, interdependent, and effective; however, they tend to be associated with underground markets and constant struggles for survival.

The administration of these social welfare programs maintains disablement and poverty as individual problems, even though the precarity born of SSI/SSDI receipt is built into the policy (see Russell 1998; Adler-Bolton and Vierkant 2020). The process of applying for and maintaining disability benefits reinforces disability identity as individualized and deficit-based. Disabled beneficiaries, therefore, are impacted personally as they experience their policy-assigned devaluation as non-contributors to the labor market. Their sense of self is often negatively impacted as they feel disregarded by society through, for example, stigmatizing comments from family, community, and benefit workers as well as through poverty-level benefits (Savin 2024).

Since the COVID-19 pandemic, despite the expansion of some social benefit programs, disabled adults living on SSI/SSDI have faced worsening poverty and material deprivation, disruptions to care routines, and additional struggles managing welfare benefits. While these harms do not often rise to the level of headlines, they have serious implications for people's ability to make ends meet and maintain a sense of self-worth. Further, they exacerbate the frequent crises born out of the precarity of disability beneficiaries' experiences as characterized by poverty, disability, rigidity, and surveillance. Too, as in other aspects of pandemic life, some of the disruptions to the normal SSI/SSDI processes improved conditions for beneficiaries.

Methods

The data were originally collected for my dissertation (2021) study entitled, *"Playing the Game" on SSI and SSDI Benefits: How Social Security Administration Policy Shapes the Individual, Societal, and Communal Disability Experience*. This is a qualitative study exploring how disabled people in California's Bay Area make ends meet on SSI/SSDI benefits and how these experiences impact beneficiaries' sense of self and identity. I interviewed 33 working-age adults (ages 18–65) using an in-depth semi-structured format. The interviews lasted anywhere from 30 minutes to two hours. After transcribing them, I used a constructivist grounded theory approach[1] to data analysis. I worked with a research assistant who also coded a portion of the interviews to add additional perspective and rigor to my analysis. Following a preliminary data analysis, I held four member-check groups in which the original participants gathered in small groups to listen to a presentation of my findings and provide feedback on any areas needing additional interpretation or emphasis. I used the qualitative and mixed methods data analysis software, Dedoose to organize the team coding process.

Framework

A Critical Disability Studies (CDS) theoretical framework guided my study. Disability is an elusive concept that moves among fissures in our society, differences in human biology and social tendencies to develop hierarchies as tools of oppression. Some CDS scholars, in recognition of these dynamic concepts, have suggested that disability be considered not an object of a lens but the lens itself; a way in which we can understand the world around us (see Minich, 2016; Kim 2016; Schalk 2017). The framework I use in this chapter emerged out of my dissertation findings and is an offshoot of Stone's (1986) political model of disability, which views disability through the lens of the political experience born out of disability as a modifiable welfare category. The administrative-, bureaucratic- and policy-defined experiences of people who fall into this category are the unifying features of the disability experience. In this model, the Social Security Model of Disability refers to the iterative process experienced by participants in which (1) SSA policy shapes society's perception of disability identity as non-participation in the workforce, (2) participants feel devalued by society at large due to their disability, and (3) participants limit their own development of families and careers in order to abide by SSA policy and maintain their benefits (Figure 4.2).

SSA's definition of disability is individualistic and medical impairment-centered, closest to the medical model of disability, and defines it in contra-distinction to participation in the labor market: "You cannot do work that you did before; We decide that you cannot adjust to other work because of your medical condition(s); and your disability has lasted or is expected to last for at least one year or to result in death" (SSA 2020) The SSA definition of disability focuses on impairments or functioning as they are related to paid work; a deficit-based understanding of disability that essentializes disabled people to their (lack of) participation and production in the labor market. Yet in describing "the poverty trap" for disabled people, Stapleton et al. (2006) note that unemployment among the disabled persists, even though "nonmedical characteristics of the individual and environment have become increasingly important to determine a person's ability to work" (710). Much of the discrimination toward disabled people stems from this conceptualization of disabled people as incapable of working and integrating into the mainstream, particularly for employers seeking effective, efficient

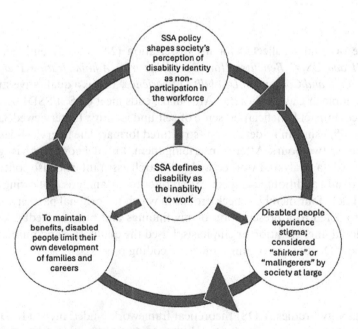

FIGURE 4.2   The Social Security Model of Disability, author.

workers.[2] In the Social Security model of disability, beneficiaries face circuitous messaging wherein their ability to obtain employment is impacted by perceptions of their employability, the need to conform to SSI/SSDI work requirements, and the provision of accommodations, in addition to any impairment-related barriers. Capacity to work is rarely a binary in lived experience as it is in policy: Some disabled people may require full-time attendant care in order to work; others may be able to work in periods between disability flare-ups; while others may be able to do certain kinds of work in particular settings or at particular times. However their impairments impact their working capacity, beneficiaries must present as unable to work to maintain eligibility for Social Security benefits. In their depiction of this process, Adler-Bolton and Vierkant (2020) explain that "labor power, social and material conditions, and bodily states are collapsed into a single metric," and disabled people must meet this myopic metric upon application and regular recertifications to survive.

The SSA's administrative characterization of disability reflects a deficit-based understanding of disabled people by defining them based on what they cannot do in an able-bodied, capitalist society. In addition to the explicit presentation of self to SSA as conforming to the agency's requirements for disability, many beneficiaries are aware that SSA can engage in surveillance of their activities to ensure the veracity of their claims, such as through the monitoring of social media, and may shift their behavior accordingly.[3] Thus, in order to access basic needs as received through the welfare state, disabled people must frequently shift their self-concept and portray their disability as a deficit rather than a cultural identity associated with pride, ingenuity, or community (Dorfman 2015). Moreover, disabled people receiving disability benefits must navigate the process of obtaining and maintaining them on their own, or in a minority of cases, with the help of a caseworker or attorney. This process reinforces the individualization of disability as a deficit that can be located within an individual rather than as a dynamic, relational, process connected to societal environments and attitudes (Chaudhry 2018; Dorfman 2017).

I analyzed this model of disability in light of my qualitative data excerpts related to COVID-19 in order to consider the overarching impact of SSA policy and how it ripples out into participants' economic capacity and decision-making, use of social safety net programs, engagement in the labor market, and sense of identity.

Findings

Findings from analysis of excerpts coded as "COVID-19" showed that the pandemic disrupted multiple areas of life, including financial management and buying power, formal and informal support systems, welfare program eligibility and management, and access to employment. Some institutional and welfare responses to the pandemic, however, provided relief to participants. I will describe each of these areas in more depth, along with an example from the data.

Worsening Poverty

Poverty plagued participants before the pandemic yet became even worse as a result of it. While people's SSI/SSDI benefit levels remained unchanged, inflation meant that the cost of basic goods such as groceries continued to increase. Living in an expensive area such as California's Bay Area on incomes as low as $783 per month requires very careful budgeting.

Further, an asset limit of $2,000 per month does not leave room for personal safety nets (SSA 2020). Even small increases in the costs of necessities caused major disruptions to participants. As one participant noted,

> Well, [COVID] has made things, it's made things be higher money-wise to pay for things—food…I'm noticing my PG&E's [Pacific Gas and Electric, a California-based gas and electric company] gone up, my rent went up, cable prices have gone up. And, you know, it's just it's making it harder for people to survive. Like right now, during the pandemic probably about three times a week, I'm missing meals.

Here, the emergency conditions brought on by the pandemic are not specific to the risk of health-related vulnerability while a highly contagious novel coronavirus circulates, but instead are a result of the exacerbation of pre-existing precarity resulting from SSI/SSDI benefit levels that started out low and remained unchanged in the face of inflation (Coleman-Jensen 2020; Coleman-Jensen and Nord 2013). Indeed, while skipping meals was a survival strategy for several participants in the post-COVID-19 interviews, some of the disabled people I interviewed prior to the pandemic also experienced food insecurity and hunger, an issue previously researched among SSI recipients (Savin et al. 2021). Lacking access to adequate nutrition is an evident health concern known to create and/or worsen medical as well as mental health issues. Thus, the experiences disabled people had because of Social Security disability program design actually produced worsening health outcomes.

In addition to rising prices that impacted people's purchasing power, participants faced added necessities not previously accounted for in their budgets, such as masks and copious amounts of hand sanitizer or other cleaning supplies. These seemingly minor items also wreaked havoc on tight budgets, requiring people to make impossible choices about what to purchase with limited funds. This type of worsening of existing poverty comes with long-lasting ripple effects:

> What kills me [is] when the account is overdrawn, and you've got to pay the overdraft fees…And then they take it out of your account at the beginning, the beginning of the month when your check comes in. You know, bye bye. And I've had that happen the last couple months because of COVID and everything.

When participants take extra funds out of their monthly benefit at the start of the month, their whole monthly budget is thrown off, throwing them into cycles of deepening scarcity that are difficult to climb out of. This participant was eventually able to borrow money from a friend, an option not available to everyone.

SSI, as a program providing income replacement for disabled people without access to the labor market, leaves its participants with little spending power, thereby contributing to illness and disability as a result of material deprivation and debility (Puar 2017). Here, *poverty acts as a mediator of health*; participants struggled to access food and basic health and protective supplies during the pandemic when these essential items were more important than ever, leaving disabled adults particularly prone to illness. For example, one participant described eating very little as a way to make ends meet, until she "wound up getting a severe case of pneumonia" from what started as a small wound and was forced to find alternative strategies. In this sense, vulnerability to COVID-19 exists separately from impairment and is instead a product of living a life dictated by Social Security policy.

Social Safety Net Disruptions

The pandemic prompted some rethinking of the US welfare state, as more people came to depend on it and thus reimagined the amount of money that might be necessary to distribute for newly unemployed people to survive. While this had short-term and (hopefully) long-term positive outcomes for welfare beneficiaries, it disrupted the rigid Social Security rules participants live with. Many participants used the housing benefit, Section 8, to access affordable housing in the expensive Bay Area on SSI/SSDI incomes. Through Section 8, people pay just 30% of their reported income toward their rent. Reporting income to Section 8 is a complex process of accounting for all of one's income and assets that is repeated on an annual basis. One participant described a nightmarish situation she faced during her annual reporting:

> They tripled my rent recently…because I got the stimulus from the government. So, they tripled my rent and ugh. So now I'm paying I'm paying my rent as it WAS before they tripled it, and I contacted the housing authority and told them. "Please lower my rent. I think you made a mistake," but…my case worker and I are waiting to hear back from the housing…I put an asterisk on it [stimulus check] and I wrote one time thing, but they took it as like the whole year. So now it's like wanting me to pay it all year, you know? I was like, oh my goodness. That's why I didn't—was scared to put [the stimulus income] on there, but I put it on there. I wanted to be straightforward with them, you know…

Here, this participant recounts the emotional and financial havoc wrecked by her receipt and required reporting of the COVID stimulus check, a universal pandemic benefit that was intended to relieve financial and emotional stress rather than create it. Over several months and with significant time, anxiety, and labor, this participant eventually was able to straighten out her rent with Section 8 through working with her case manager to contact Section 8 and file the appropriate appeals. However, she risked her housing in the process since she was unable to afford the inappropriately raised rent and feared that her landlord would evict her. The benefit of the stimulus check was quickly counteracted by the panic and expense of the ordeal. This type of situation is repeated with other pandemic-related changes to people's budgets, as any minor change to a system that has both rigid rules and inefficient bureaucracy could create barriers to benefit receipt. While the stimulus checks were largely beneficial to SSI/SSDI beneficiaries and the idea of universal cash transfers is a welcome alternative to the current welfare model, the ensuing problems underscored the crisis-prone nature resulting from the degree of surveillance and rigidity with which beneficiaries live.

Informal Survival Strategies Upended

In part to cope with this surveillance and rigidity, some participants managed to make ends meet through informal survival strategies outside of the safety net system. These often included engaging in underground economies, bartering, trading with other SSI/SSDI recipients, and making use of personal connections to access free or low-cost necessities. The disruptions to everyday life brought on by the COVID-19 pandemic altered everyone's context for living, which included the context of participants' informal, creative workarounds. For example, one participant described the local practice of acquiring home goods and clothing through a semi-annual Berkeley event: Students moving in and out of dorm rooms and leaving items they no longer wanted on the street.

It's called Hippy Christmas or Hobo Christmas, Bums' Christmas... And it happens, you know, twice a year. And. Well, the thing is, you know, students throw away some crazy stuff. So, the really adventurous folks...they do all the dumpster diving and stuff like that. And find for, you know, phones and laptops and all this stuff that's thrown away in a frenzy to get out and get home. And weed. I mean, crazy stuff. And so... mostly I just get clothes and look out for kitchen supplies... I have an awesome cast iron Dutch oven you know, stuff like that. That's my thing. But the university stopped allowing students to place items outside this year.

In an effort to prevent students from mingling outside of campus dorms during the hectic move-out season and potentially spreading COVID-19, the university implemented new policies requiring students to register with a private service that would remove unwanted items from dorm rooms, thus canceling Hobo Christmas. This participant described having to add clothing and miscellaneous home goods back into her budget which created ripple effects that strained an already tight budget. The lack of interaction with the community more broadly during the start of the COVID-19 pandemic hampered participants' abilities to participate in their economies, which were rooted in hard cash and trades of physical items that could escape the SSA oversight of banking systems and electronic cash transfers.

Increased Employment Discrimination

Many participants supplemented their cash benefits with part-time work, both under and over the table. For the two participants whose work became remote, they found access much improved and described having wanted to work remotely for years with their requests to do so previously having been denied. However, most participants who worked found their jobs eliminated due to pandemic restrictions and struggled to find new work in the newly tightened job market. One participant expressed significant distress over her newly unemployed status, as she was a mother to three young children and unable to find new work:

It's been challenging because I can't find a job that will accommodate my disability and keep myself safe. And without, you know, I mean, there's no availability of jobs right now for someone who's on Social Security disability... because we are a compromise ... everything is limited, especially right now in the pandemic. There are so many people that need to work from home. So, I didn't think that I even had a chance. And, you know, that really affected me for my self-esteem down and my confidence down.

In a devastating turn of phrase, this participant described her perception of how employers think about hiring disabled employees: As a compromise. Previously in the interview, she discussed her need for accommodations in the workplace as well as the SSDI policy that prohibits her from earning more per month than the amount deemed by SSA as Substantial Gainful Activity—$1,260 for non-blind individuals in 2020 (SSA 2020). Her rigid cap on hours she could work each month on top of her need for physical accommodation, she presumed, made her less desirable as an employee than a non-disabled person not tied to benefit-related income restrictions.

As a Black, disabled, woman receiving SSDI, this participant faced multiple types of workplace discrimination. This was the first extended period of unemployment she experienced since she was a teenager, and she was left devastated financially as well as existentially—especially given the larger meaning she made of her inability to work. She was not alone as many participants described how the impacts of living under SSA policy impacted their psyches: "You feel like you're inferior to other people... like I must be different from everyone else... and as we've said, they [SSA] have a very narrow definition of it [disability]." While disabled people have always faced employment discrimination, they were particularly impacted by employment conditions in the first year of the pandemic, as they perceived that the few jobs available would go to non-disabled workers before them. This perception was rooted both in blatant employer discrimination faced by participants with apparent disabilities as well as those whose disabilities were not apparent but had to negotiate their work hours with their employer based on SSA-imposed limits to monthly earnings. In fact, the need to disclose these SSA-imposed work limitations rendered disabilities apparent. Here, the Social Security Model of Disability operated on multiple levels, as participants had to out themselves as disabled in their discussion of work limitations that originated in SSA policy rather than individual impairment. This served to *further conflate the state of being disabled with an inability to work* and forced participants to limit their own career development and capacity for earning.

Improvements

Not everything about the COVID-19 pandemic worsened conditions for disabled SSI/SSDI beneficiaries in the Bay Area. Disabled people vary in their disabilities and necessary accommodations, so it is no surprise that some changing conditions related to COVID-19 benefited some participants. Consider the pivot to online and tele-services instead of in-person interactions. The Social Security Administration closed its physical offices at the start of the COVID-19 pandemic and began allowing SSI recipients to conduct business online. For example, those on SSI engaging in any work activity previously had to submit their pay stubs for any paychecks during the month it was received at an SSA office. This was challenging for those with mobility disabilities in particular, since this meant finding time during the work week in normal business hours to get to an office, rather than using the necessary transportation resources to go to work. Participants also reported being able to have many types of appointments with SSA workers by phone, as it not only spared them the burden of travel but also the often stigmatizing and tiring experience of waiting to be seen in an SSA office that is characteristic of the Social Security Model of disability. Yet for some participants, particularly those with cognitive and developmental disabilities, navigating online portals was confusing and more stressful than in-person interactions. This suggests that people with disabilities would benefit from the maintenance of both options of in-person and remote social services delivery and benefit coordination.

Some resources that supported participants were expanded at the start of the COVID-19 pandemic to account for the added hardship brought on by the pandemic. However, for many participants, the increase in resources and added benefits were long-awaited from their already dire circumstances. Thus, they were needed sooner and will be needed after the time-limited expansions. For example, CalFresh benefits, which are California's Supplemental Nutritional Assistance Program benefits (colloquially referred to as food stamps), increased for all recipients from amounts as low as $12 per month to the maximum allotment of $194 for an individual in 2020. CalFresh has continued to increase over the last couple of years to account for ongoing pandemic-related food insecurity and inflation.

In addition to increasing benefit generosity, CalFresh and other welfare programs eased the burden of participation. For example, CalFresh provided six-month extensions for benefit recertification and those receiving Section 8 housing benefits found that workers skipped their routine home visits that some participants experienced as invasive and a form of government surveillance. Additionally, federal policy paused the recertification requirement for Medicaid, allowing for continuous health coverage during the pandemic. In addition to improving program participation rates, reductions to administrative burden such as these can have significant benefits to beneficiaries' overall well-being in their capacity to reduce welfare-related stigma.

Discussion

Participants' experiences of both struggle and relative ease during the COVID-19 pandemic are valuable simply as documentation of lives that are often overlooked and lacking in political power. Further, their capacities to make ends meet during the crises of daily life and during a global pandemic are instructive for welfare policy and programmatic decision-making that can address the reality of how policies are lived in quotidian disabled life. The pandemic's increased ease in access to benefits and their greater generosity, unsurprisingly, are policies that enhanced the food security and overall stability of disabled people's lives. These benefit increases took on greater salience in the setting of social isolation in which participants' use of community and creative economic structures were often unavailable to them, hence worsening existing precarity. While these informal mechanisms of making ends meet are not typically accounted for in policy assessments of SSI/SSDI beneficiary income amounts, they were a critical part of participants' own budgeting, particularly those on SSI.

On an organizational level, programs that provide home delivery of food aid to older adults such as Meals on Wheels, as opposed to most food banks that require transportation to access, could be expanded to serve disabled people who also face transportation access barriers. Some study participants noted that they looked for these programs but found that as disabled people under age 65, they were not eligible. Further, localities could add home delivery options for food banks to increase access to disabled people, particularly during emergency conditions such as a pandemic when vulnerability to infection increases transportation barriers. Food banks might also be used as sites that provide other essentials of daily living necessary, such as toiletries and PPE, that help maintain health.

People on SSI/SSDI who live in high cost of living regions, such as California's Bay Area, must rely on multiple forms of welfare in order to make ends meet, which means that they are typically navigating programmatic guidelines at multiple levels of government including county (e.g., In Home Support Services), state (e.g., CalFresh), and federal (e.g., SSI) levels. When all programs are means-tested such as in these examples and programs are not in coordination with each other due to differing administrative bodies, participants risk being kicked off. While in the long term, enhanced coordination among these programs is needed, in the short term, it is crucial to enact policies that pause means-testing and recertification requirements during emergency conditions. Further, any local or organizational efforts to provide financial support to individuals during crisis periods might consider using gift cards or visa cards to avoid impacting cash benefits of SSI/SSDI recipients.

This balancing act that a beneficiary must navigate in SSI/DI became so ingrained in some participants that it further shaped their sense of self under the Social Security model. This constant psychic work of assessing one's finances that may be surveilled, managing paperwork for various programs, and abiding by multiple sets of benefit conditions is a feature of the model. Exploring ways to ease this balancing act may serve dual purposes: A form of practical relief for essential goods and services as well as relief to the chronic anxiety and the cognitive labor of managing benefits.

Conclusion

Participants' pandemic experiences of finances, employment, care, and sense of self can largely be traced back to the influence of SSA's model of disability that persists across officially declared emergency conditions and de facto emergency conditions. Both participants' areas of increased struggle and relative ease of access illustrate the highly precarious, untenable nature of their daily lives. The ripple effects of near or below poverty-level benefits exacerbate the experience of inflationary prices and new costly routines required to survive the COVID-19 pandemic. Further, the inability of SSI recipients to maintain any type of personal safety net through the $2k asset limit leaves them even more vulnerable to any shifts in budget management. Both factors—low benefits and low assets—necessitate the use of multiple welfare programs to cover various life expenses. Although welfare programs such as SSI and CalFresh do help in making ends meet, they are in many cases insufficient and add additional rigid guidelines and complex bureaucracy to navigate. While the COVID-19 pandemic was an opportunity to create the political will to improve, even if temporarily, some welfare-related conditions for disabled participants, the enhancements must continue and be expanded upon to build a safety net that can alleviate poverty and hunger before, during, and after officially recognized emergency conditions. This is particularly salient given the ongoing nature of precarity and vulnerability to crisis that disabled communities impacted by the SSA model of disability experience.

Acknowledgments

This chapter was based on data originally collected for my dissertation, which was supported by: (1) The Institute for Research on Labor and Employment at University of California Berkeley and (2) Policy Research, Inc. which requires the following disclosure: *the research reported herein was performed pursuant to a grant from Policy Research, Inc. as part of the US Social Security Administration's (SSA's) Analyzing Relationships Between Disability, Rehabilitation and Work. The opinions and conclusions expressed are solely those of the author(s) and do not represent the opinions or policy of Policy Research, Inc., SSA or any other agency of the Federal Government.* This chapter benefited from the edits and thoughtful feedback of the editors for which I am grateful.

Notes

1 Constructivist grounded theory, rooted in an interpretative tradition, contrasts itself with objectivist grounded theory through perceiving the data collection and analysis process as a social action, or construction, that is co-created among study participants and researchers. Thus, unlike in positivist research where researcher bias is assumed to be fully eliminated, the researcher's perspective and values are assumed to be non-neutral and to shape the study findings (Charmaz 2014).

2 This discrimination may also be correlated to disability hate, as documented in Sherry 2016; Jammaers, Zanoni, and Hardonk 2016.

3 See (SSA 2019, 26) for description of SSA's use of social media in the disability determination process.

Works Cited

Adler-Bolton, Beatrice, and Artie Vierkant. 2020. *Health Communism: A Surplus Manifesto*. Brooklyn, NY: Verso.

Center on Budget and Policy Priorities. 2022 "Policy Basics: Supplemental Security Income." August 12, 2022. https://www.cbpp.org/research/social-security/supplemental-security-income

Charmaz, Kathy. 2014. *Constructing Grounded Theory*. Thousand Oaks, CA: Sage.

Chaudhry, Vandana. 2018. "Knowing through tripping: A performative praxis for co constructing knowledge as a disabled halfie." *Qualitative Inquiry* 24 (1): 70–82.

Coleman-Jensen, Alisha. 2020. "US food insecurity and population trends with a focus on adults with disabilities." *Physiology & Behavior* 220: 112865.

Coleman-Jensen, Alisha and Mark Nord. 2013. "Disability Is an Important Risk Factor for Food Insecurity." *USDA Economic Research Service*, May 6, 2013. https://www.ers.usda.gov/amber-waves/2013/may/disability-is-an-important-risk-factor-for-food-insecurity

Dorfman, Doron. 2015. "Disability Identity in Conflict: Performativity in the US Social Security Benefits System." *Thomas Jefferson Law Review* 38: 47.

Dorfman, Doron. 2017. "Re-claiming Disability: Identity, Procedural Justice, and the Disability Determination Process." *Law & Social Inquiry* 42 (1): 195–231.

Goodley, Dan, Rebecca Lawthom, and Katherine Runswick-Cole. 2014. "Dis/Ability and Austerity: Beyond Work and Slow Death." *Disability & Society* 29 (6): 980–984. https://doi.org/10.1080/09687599.2014.920125

Jammaers, Eline, Patrizia Zanoni, and Stefan Hardonk. 2016. "Constructing Positive Identities in Ableist Workplaces: Disabled employees' Discursive Practices Engaging with the Discourse of Lower Productivity." *Human Relations* 69 (6): 1365–1386.

Kim, Jina B. 2016. "Toward a Crip-of-Color Critique: Thinking with Minich's 'Enabling Whom?'" *Lateral* 6 (1). https://doi.org/10.25158/L6.1.14

Minich, J. 2016. "Enabling Whom? Critical Disability Studies Now." *Lateral* 5 (1). https://doi.org/10.25158/L5.1.9

Puar, Jasbir K. 2017. *The Right to Maim: Debility, Capacity, Disability*. Durham, NC: Duke University Press.

Russell, Marta. 1998. *Beyond Ramps: Disability at the End of the Social Contract: A Warning from an Uppity Crip*. Monroe, ME: Common Courage Press.

Savin, Katie, Alena Morales, Ronli Levi, Dora Alvarez, and Hilary Seligman. 2021. "'Now I Feel a Little Bit More Secure': The Impact of SNAP Enrollment on Older Adult SSI Recipients." *Nutrients* 13 (12): 4362.

Savin, Katie. 2024. ""Everyone Else Gets to Have the American Dream:" How Social Security Disability Policy Shapes Disability Identity." *Journal of Sociology and Social Welfare* 51 (1). https://doi.org/10.15453/0191-5096.4736

Schalk, Sami. 2017. "Critical Disability Studies as Methodology." *Lateral* 6 (1). https://doi.org/10.25158/L6.1.13

Sherry, Mark. 2016. *Disability Hate Crimes: Does Anyone Really Hate Disabled People?* New York: Routledge.

Social Security Administration. 2019. *Fiscal Year 2020 Budget Overview*. Washington, DC: Social Security Administration. https://www.ssa.gov/budget/assets/materials/2018/2018BO.pdf

Social Security Administration. 2020. *The Red Book - A Guide to Work Incentives*. Washington, DC: Social Security Administration. https://www.ssa.gov/redbook/

Stapleton, David C., Bonnie L. O'Day, Gina A. Livermore, and Andrew J. Imparato. 2006. "Dismantling the Poverty Trap: Disability Policy for the Twenty-first Century." *The Milbank Quarterly* 84 (4): 701–732.

Stone, Deborah A. 1986. *The Disabled State*. Philadelphia, PA: Temple University Press.

5

CHRONIC INJUSTICE

Racialized Disablement and the Urgency of the Everyday

Desiree Valentine

Analysis of the emergency conditions of the pandemic urges renewed attention to the underlying facets of society that have deepened the pandemic's harms—those structural elements of society that create, perpetuate, maintain, and extend injury, illness, and disease through resource allocation procedures, social and political disenfranchisement, geopolitical and punitive containment practices, environmental toxicities, and state violence. Scholars have referred to this phenomenon in a variety of ways—disablement (2002), debilitation (Puar 2017), and emergent disability (Ribet 2011), to name a few. In this chapter, I show how the sociopolitical production and infliction of disablement operate through a temporality of *chronic injustice*. That is, harms perpetuated by the state serve as the persistent background in which episodes of exceptional violence reoccur, thereby further entrenching ongoing violence. We can see this perhaps most clearly in the history and political situation of racially marginalized individuals who face disablement by the state in myriad forms. As this chapter argues, we must attend to both the exceptionality and mundanity of state-supported harm against marginalized populations to better prevent and address conditions of persistent and often invisibilized crisis.

I begin by outlining how scholars have theorized the sociopolitical production of disability. I then describe how the chronicity of injustice depends upon oppressive norms and practices surrounding what constitutes states of "emergency" and "normality." As I show, the contours of these terms are maintained through the continued production of populations as *expendable*. This results in the maintenance of the status quo and an exculpation of state responsibility for further harms inflicted upon populations. Next, I examine the intersection of processes of racialization and disablement in both the immediate conditions of the pandemic and the long duration of injustices perpetuated against racialized communities. The intertwinement of systems of racism and ableism generates what I call *racialized disablement*. I argue that we ought to understand "race" and "disability" in their simultaneity in order to best confront the chronicity of injustice that faces us.

DOI: 10.4324/9781003502623-8

The Sociopolitical Production of Disability

The COVID-19 pandemic is one of the largest and clearest expressions of the multifarious ways in which disability is a sociopolitical production. Disability can be identified as a socio-political production when "physical, cognitive, and/or psychological conditions are wholly or partially caused by social inequity," oftentimes "grounded in class and economics, gender, sexuality, race, ethnicity, immigration, status, age, or other disabilities," and oftentimes oper-ating "at the intersection of several of these demographics simultaneously" (Ribet 2011, 161). Legal scholar Beth Ribet refers to this as "emergent disability," a subset of the broader cate-gory of disability that includes the *inflicted* experience of injury as opposed to genetic condi-tions, normative aging processes, and accidents of circumstance (2011, 161–62). Emergent disabilities can be caused by workplace safety violations, the spread of environmental toxins, cuts to welfare, and lack of healthcare. It is in part *because* of already ongoing oppressions and concomitant processes of disablement that the effects of the pandemic have impacted certain communities so deeply. For many poor, disabled, Black, Indigenous, Latinx, and other people of color, the threat of COVID-19 arose amidst harmful work environments, the dwin-dling of welfare services, and inaccessible and low-quality healthcare. Instead of experiencing the pandemic as an exceptional crisis, for many it was an extension and compounding of state-sanctioned violence in the form of ongoing exploitation, neglect, and abandonment.

It is likely that emergent disability comprises a substantial portion of the disabled popula-tion, yet it is rarely foregrounded in disability analysis. As Ribet writes, "while disability-based subordination is recognized as a social phenomenon, there is often no integrated political attention to why disability manifests in particular individuals or communities" (2011, 160). There is however a sustained and growing body of literature within critical disability studies that stands as an exception to this. Early discussions of the political production of disable-ment focused on the intersection of capitalism and disability. Scholars have importantly iden-tified how capitalism necessitates the category of "disabled" for those who cannot participate in the capitalist mandate for productivity and then deems such people "unproductive" and therefore (implicitly or explicitly) less worthy of care and concern in a market economy (Russell 2019; Russell and Stewart 2001; Oliver and Barnes 2012. Moreover, these scholars have interrogated how industrial capitalism and "productivity at any cost" generated "dis-abling accidents and conditions...at an unprecedented rate" (Russell and Stewart 2001). A materialist analysis of disability, they argued, was necessary to move beyond a mere rights or recognition discourse that served mainly to include some—more privileged disabled indi-viduals—into a system that generated social and material exclusion for many.

More recent discussions of the sociopolitical production of disablement are oriented by the transnational turn in disability studies (Gary, 2021). Scholars have studied the ways in which disablement for certain populations is often not understood *as disability*, but unfortu-nate side effects of culture or bad moral luck (Puar 2017; Erevelles 2011; McRuer 2018; Gorman 2016). This includes populations such as those of the global south, those undergo-ing state conflict and apartheid, and those who are negatively racialized and/or impover-ished. Jasbir K. Puar has interrogated how state processes generate disablement by focusing on *debilitation*. As she writes, debilitation refers to the "slow wearing down of populations." With this, she describes "debility" as the "triangulation of the ability/disability binary," and asks what drops out of frame given the "racialization of bodies that are expected to endure pain, suffering, and injury" (Puar 2017, xiv). By introducing the term debilitation to the conversation related to disability, Puar brings attention to the mechanisms by which disablement is a *process* that is often made invisible by a network of social norms, policy, and direct state violence.

Work on the relation between capitalism and disability and the global, transnational study of disability involves analysis of the fluidity of disability as a concept—who it attaches to and how—and the role of the state. These areas of inquiry embrace an approach to disability studies that is primarily concerned with what disability *does* as a concept, as a relationship, and as an experience and how this "doing" operates on discursive, embodied, interpersonal, and structural levels. They also employ the distinction between the state as benevolent protector of disability rights versus the state as inflictor of (slow or immediate) violence that disables populations. Increasingly, the state recognizes "the disabled" as "those whose formal relationship to the state enables them to claim benefits, while others with similar embodied experiences continue to work through injury and illness or languish without benefits or status" (Gorman 2016, 254). We might think here of immigrants, impoverished individuals, and those negatively racialized or deemed a foreigner. Dominant understandings of the state as solely protector and enforcer of disability rights obscures its own role in producing or neglecting to prevent disablement via its economic and political systems, labor processes, and mechanisms of social stratification, such as race, citizenship, and nationality.

Much is at stake in how we recognize disability, especially in terms of the positioning of the state. The state inflicts and allows the generation of disability while maintaining the cover of supposed protector, but only for select classes of people. The infliction of disability is made invisible through the persistence of attitudes, norms, values, and practices that position injury, illness, and disablement of certain populations (impoverished, racialized, immigrant, etc.) as culturally or biologically justified, rather than as an effect of wrongful state actions.

We must therefore continue to ask: when does disability emerge as a possible identity that confers rights and protections and when is disablement rendered justification for continued neglect or abuse? Processes of racialization, impoverishment, exploitation, and other forms of marginalization are key to answering this question. The sociopolitical production of disablement involves both the literal production of mental and physical disabilities (the resultant "emergent disability") as well as the interpretive work of determining who "counts" as disabled and why or how. While disability is often used as a category to describe a state of being, it is also and perhaps more foundationally, a *system* and *process*—with both material and discursive dimensions. In the sections to follow, I explore the phenomenon of the sociopolitical production of disability via its concomitant temporal conditions and then consider how racialization and disablement processes function together.

Injustice as Chronic: Emergency, Normalcy, and Who Matters

Conditions of "emergency" and "normalcy" are privileged positions for a select class of individuals while many live in states of what we might call chronic injustice. Chronic injustice names the longstanding dynamics of institutions, built environments, corporations, governments, and social mores that inflict wrongful harms. It is persistent and engrained and therefore requires attention to a lengthy historiography and deep meditation on the social and political undercurrents of the nation and broader society. Instead of narrowing in on the specific and immediate dynamics of the pandemic, understanding injustice as chronic points us to the background conditions and histories that propel and exacerbate the present situations in which we find ourselves. Developing a broader and deeper historical and socio-political analysis of "emergency" conditions better positions us to prevent harms in the future and mediate the accumulated harms in the present.

From slavery and colonization to residential schools and Jim Crow, to criminalization and pathologization of marginalized racial, classed, and gendered populations, grave injustices span our history. These injustices are state-manufactured phenomena that produce disabling conditions for certain populations and then pose these as a natural and normative feature of society. Take for instance the following historical example. First published in 1920, W.E.B. Du Bois' literary text *Darkwater: Voices from within the Veil* inventories the violences of white-ness, lynching, war, capitalism, and more. Saidiya Hartman, reflecting on this text 100 years later in the early stages of the COVID-19 pandemic, writes:

> The influenza pandemic of 1918 does not appear in [Du Bois'] inventory. Perhaps because microbes seemed benign when compared with the bloodletting of the Red Summer. Or because every year between 1906 and 1920, black folks in cities experienced a rate of death that equaled the white rate of death at the peak of the pandemic. When the Spanish influ-enza arrived, *they simply died in even greater numbers*, but they had been enduring a pan-demic for over a decade. Du Bois resisted the impulse to calculate comparative mortality or produce a death table because it was all too obvious. He knew that the facts of blackness, the statistics, the mathematical equation, and the calculations of probability would not change anything. *They had been allowed to die in great numbers without a crisis ever being declared.*
>
> *(2020, emphasis mine)*

Hartman's reflection urges us to investigate the meanings of "emergency" and "normalcy" and the function of expendability amid conditions of chronic injustice. Prior to the pandemic, there was no "crisis" declared concerning the chronic injustices associated with simply being a poor, racialized, disabled, and/or chronically ill person in a society structured by oppression. Rather, this was simply deemed a normal, or perhaps *normative*, way of life for many.

As many might recall, almost immediately after the pandemic was first declared an emer-gency in the United States in March 2020, there were calls from elected officials, economists, and others that we need to "get back to normal." These calls were coupled specifically with the awareness that Black, Brown, poor, disabled, incarcerated, and those with chronic condi-tions and in nursing homes were experiencing transmission, hospitalization, and death at much higher rates. The continued rush to "get back to normal" was made through the implicit and sometimes explicit acceptance of certain populations as "disposable." Indeed, some offi-cials openly promoted the idea that elderly and disabled people were expendable and that their "preventable deaths were preferable to a slowed-down economy" (Pulrang 2021).

Populations deemed disposable have also often then become identified as the locus of or even the *culprit* for their own deaths. Early in the pandemic social media posts began circulat-ing suggesting that only 6% of COVID-19-related deaths were from COVID-19 because the additional 94% of deaths were listed as cases of comorbidity wherein COVID-19 was listed as one cause of death among others, such as pneumonia, diabetes, obesity, and respiratory fail-ure (Reuters 2020). The push to enumerate the rates by which individuals were affected according to co-emergent conditions was done in order to downplay the effects of the virus and to suggest that it wasn't *COVID-19* that caused death in these populations, but underlying illness and by extension, already-ill populations *themselves*. We see a similar pattern emerge in cases of police murders of Black and Brown individuals wherein testimony of pre-existing health conditions of the victim is used to try and exculpate murderous acts, such as kneeling on someone's neck for nearly nine minutes or suffocating one using an illegal chokehold. Ann Crawford-Roberts et al. describe this as the "weaponization of medical language reinforc[ing] white supremacy" (Ann Crawford-Roberts et al. 2020).

These examples make clear how the scope of one's moral and political community is shaped by what is deemed "normal" and what is deemed an "emergency." A situation becomes an emergency when it impacts those who have yet to be impacted or who have yet to be impacted to the degree to which others are "normally" impacted. This calculation bears on our societal practices of evaluating how care, access, and intervention procedures should be handled. "Emergency" seems to be reserved for the protection of the dominant class. That is, the dominant paradigm of "emergency" signals a state of exception, something that, in its catastrophic destruction, reaches states of affairs outside the "norm" of acceptability or sustainability. The dark underside of this, however, is that the abundance of chronic injustices facing myriad populations is reinforced as *acceptable* and even *required* for the status quo to remain. Take for example the irony that it was the "municipal *Emergency Manager*" in Flint, Michigan, that, in the interest of "financial solvency" decided to change the city's water supply to Lake Huron and have the—overwhelmingly poor and people of color—of Flint to "absorb the costs of infrastructure (unrepaired), deindustrialization (which moved wealth elsewhere) and financialization (in the form of laws privileging bond holders above all others) in their bodies" (Jampel 2018, 8). He who was tasked with "managing" emergency instead created a *genuine emergency* that would go unrecognized, while the management of emergency affecting the elite was prioritized.

As we see here, the politics of naming crisis situations ultimately relies on a politics of naming who is worthy of care and who is expendable and thus grievable. As the Health Care Access Sub-committee of the COVID-19 Working Group of New York highlights: "If anything is 'normal,' it is the very human realities of illness and disability across the life span; it is the disabling structures of society that isolate and disregard those among us who are living with them" (COVID-19 Working Group of New York 2020). Indeed, what has been normal is the persistence of disabling conditions generated by a lack of material and social infrastructure, antiblack racism, and poverty: at base, the persistent and organized *extraction from* and *abandonment of* racialized, disabled, and impoverished populations.

Opposed to dominant paradigms of interpreting normalcy and emergency that maintain a harmful status quo for marginalized individuals, critical studies of race, disability, and poverty illuminate how conditions of "normalcy" are ongoing *conditions of emergency* experienced by many Black, Brown, poor, disabled, and chronically ill individuals. Such experiences are naturalized as emergent from and contained in the bodies of individuals when they are anything but.

When analyzing the social and political production of disablement and illness, it is thus important to reframe chronic conditions as chronic *injustices*. The concentration of harm in certain populations is not "natural" but an effect of dominant power systems that accumulate and compound harm across generations. Understanding how chronic injustice configures the sociopolitical production of disablement and vice versa allows us to 1) bear witness to the *unnaturalness* of many of the effects of the pandemic; 2) name societal actors and conditions that produce the compounded effects of harm on marginalized populations; and 3) seek redress and societal change to alleviate those effects. In what follows, I offer a conceptual intervention into how we understand the relation between processes of racialization and disablement that is spurred by awareness of the sociopolitical production of disablement and the temporality of injustice.

Racialized Disablement: Racism, Ableism, and the Pandemic

In this section, I offer the concept of racialized disablement as a heuristic for understanding race and disability as co-articulating social markers and racism and ableism as fundamentally entangled social systems. There are two key reasons for developing the concept of racialized disablement in the way that I do: First, to demonstrate the need for a conceptual confrontation—or what I call a method of juxtaposition—between "race" and "disability" and second, to capture the endurance and depth of intertwined processes of racism and ableism. Understanding racialized disablement in this way helps us reframe interpretations of the conditions leading up to the pandemic, the experiences therein, and the effects of the pandemic on racialized populations. Additionally, it provides a language for identifying wrongful actions and societal conditions as well as preventing the accumulation of harms in the future. I begin by discussing the intersection of ableism of racism, both in theory and practice, which then leads to my discussion of racialized disablement as a conceptual tool.

The Ableism and Racism Structuring the Pandemic

Like many other crises to come before, the COVID pandemic did not impact all those who experienced it equally. Indeed, as has become wildly clear, the harms of the pandemic have disproportionately affected Black and Brown populations on a greater scale and in more complex ways given our historical inheritances as a society. Take the case of housing discrimination against African Americans over the last century, which has produced obstacles for home ownership and forced many individuals into rental or intergenerational housing situations. The initial lockdowns produced especially difficult living situations and quarantine procedures for these housing types. We can add to this the fact that many "essential workers," especially those in transportation services who had high contact with the public, were Black and Brown, low-income folks (McNicholas and Poydock 2020). Beyond the immediate threat of illness from the virus, the intersection of racist housing and economic discrimination produced countless issues relating to care for family members, housing and economic insecurity, and eviction concerns.

Black folks also faced harms related to deeply engrained patterns of racism in interpersonal interactions with nurses and physicians. Consider the heart-wrenching case of Susan Moore, a Black medical doctor who was hospitalized in the early days of the pandemic. As Moore sought treatment based on her own knowledge as a physician, she faced resistance from her white medical doctor who expressed discomfort in giving her more narcotics and who subsequently discharged her. Just two weeks later, Moore died from complications related to COVID. In a video posted to Facebook, Moore detailed the inadequacy of care and disrespect she felt while in the hospital. As she describes, "[The doctor] made me feel like a drug addict...I put forth and maintain that if I was white, I wouldn't have to go through that" (Elingon 2020). There is a long and documented history of doctors downplaying Black individuals' pain from slavery onward. It is this duration of engrained social mores that contributes not only to racist interactions, but significant health and disability consequences including death.

Furthermore, a 2022 study showed that White individuals' awareness of COVID-19 racial disparities predicted *reduced* support for COVID safety precautions, suggesting that White individuals felt less inclined to work to collectively prevent COVID when rates of transmission, disease, and death were highest in marginalized populations (Skinner-Dorkeno et al. 2022). That is, white individuals felt *less* moved to address pandemic concerns when provided with the knowledge that COVID was more heavily affecting populations already deemed disposable. So, it is not only the case that COVID itself generated compounded effects for racialized populations, but that white supremacy—or what some have called a fundamental *racial value gap* that presupposes white people as more valuable than others—generated a further accumulation of disease and disablement for such populations.[1] Therefore, it is not simply the case that poverty or race are forms of social stratification that make one more susceptible to disablement, but that white supremacy is *indebted* to (or perhaps necessarily coupled with) a system of abled normativity wherein disablement is *expected* to concentrate in certain communities.[2] The construction of abled normativity becomes co-extensive with whiteness and constitutive of black *disability* and disablement.

The effects of this intersection between white supremacy and ableism accumulate and compound *across time*. Prior to the pandemic, Black individuals in the United States lived with higher rates of high blood pressure, diabetes, and heart disease, in part because of stressors related to racism. When the pandemic hit, many of these conditions placed Black individuals at higher risk for complications from COVID. Here we see the physiological harms of racism as compounded by the acute effects of COVID and all this amid the temporal backdrop of continued injustices—police brutality, worker harms, lack of welfare supports, and more.

Scholars and activists have thus incisively referred to COVID-19 and ongoing state harm and violence against Black Americans as "twin pandemics" (Beesley 2020; McCarty 2020; Moore and Gray-Garcia 2020; National Academy of Medicine 2020; Santa Clara University 2020). As Rinaldo Walcott (2020) writes, "the catastrophe of COVID-19 resides in an already existing state-derived practice of antiblack racism" (158). Harkening back to Du Bois' recognition of the violence against Black Americans which was occurring long before (and then alongside) the harms wrought by the 1918 pandemic, this line of thinking urges us to not only name these two phenomena as concurrent but theorize their mutually constitutive intertwinement. As Ersula J. Ore puts it: "Breathing in times of suffocating anti-blackness demands recognition that the degree of difference between Breonna Taylor, Ahmaud Arbery, George Floyd, and the…Black victims of COVID-19 is marginal; it is a difference of form, not motive" (Chirindo et al. 2020, 462). The underlying disabling motive remains clear across time, space, and history and it is this phenomenon I wish to bring to the fore through the terminology of *racialized disablement*.

Racialized Disablement as Conceptual Tool

It should be clear at this point how the sustained patterns of racism and ableism both prior to and during the pandemic have generated a phenomenon which calls for attention and repair. The way in which this intersection is made invisible by being cast as natural or normal is one way it continues. To prevent the scale and form of such crises in the future, we need to illuminate these temporal and sociopolitical dimensions and develop conceptual tools to address their harms.

The concept of *racialized disablement* forces a juxtaposition between "race" and "disability" and "racism" and "ableism," challenging their presumed discreteness and urging inquiry into how our sociopolitical order is actively organized to make opaque the conditions leading up to, as well as the actors involved in, the generation of harm.[3] Juxtaposition requires us to place two seemingly distinct items next to one another and view them simultaneously such that our awareness and understanding of each is transformed in the process. The role of juxtaposition is to create an *effect*. In this case, the intended effect is a hesitation at and rethinking of the analytical separation of race and disability, of racism and ableism, across history and contemporarily. The *goal* of this method of inquiry is to 1) bear witness to the sociopolitical *production* of race and disability at the site of what I call racialized disablement, 2) name relevant social actors such as the state, corporations, policies, etc. in generating and compounding disablement and 3) reorient responses to these harms—moving from cultural or genetic deterministic evaluations to social, political, and ethical commitments to repair.

"Racialized disablement" aims to forge a more thorough awareness of how race and disability *function*. Using more process-based terms related to the social markers "race" and "disability," we can heighten the sense in which both are not neutral descriptors that pertain to individual bodies, but rather persist in contexts of ongoing structural oppressions. Ultimately, racialized disablement is a strategy of interpretation, accounting for, and making sense of oppressions as they rely on and structure one another, producing racial disparities in health, inequities in civic inclusion, and violent power dynamics in law, policy, and criminal punishment.[4]

Racialized disablement captures how racism and ableism are not past historical or singular events but are ongoing co-constitutive systems of power—historically, politically, and conceptually intertwined. These oppressive social systems rely on one another to carry out aims of marginalization, exploitation, and neglect. And they require one another to function *as* racism or *as* ableism. What I mean by this is that racism and ableism are so deeply ingrained into our fundamental terms, concepts, and modern ways of practicing and understanding what it means to be human that they are inseparable. Theorists have worked to describe how racism and ableism are not additive or parallel oppressions, but deeply rooted in and dependent on one another. My interpretation of the relation between racism and ableism is aligned with work committed to thinking about their rooted entanglement and in ways that illuminate and clarify our histories and present states.

Opposed to a narrow definition of ableism as the set of values and/or practices that discriminate against and devalue disabled bodies and minds, writer and activist Talila 'TL' Lewis (2023) identifies ableism as a more fundamental and organizing oppressive force whose "categorization/ranking/valuation of bodyminds" provides the mechanism and support for myriad oppressions. Ableism, according to Lewis, defines bodyminds, behaviors, or community characteristics as "inferior or superior, unworthy or worthy, useless or useful, normative or deviant, etc." Given the context of the United States, "these valuations and rankings are in/formed through the application of white supremacist settler-colonial cisheteropatriarchal capitalist ideas about race, ethnicity, dis/ability, gender, re/productivity, criminality, civility, intelligence, fitness, beauty, birth/living place, etc."

Racism, too, is a system through which our social markers and experiences are fundamentally shaped. As various scholars have argued, the "human" in modernity is founded on the racial and so "racial violence is always/already internal to humanising discourses" (Gorman

2016, 257). What it means to be "human" itself is racially coded and filtered through racial/racist discourses and violences (Weheliye 2014). As Joel M. Reynolds (2022) argues, the institution and persistence of white supremacy involve "a process of *making abled and disabled*" (50). White supremacy organizes the world by generating abilities, or markers that identify privileges for some groups at the expense of others. This has historically involved landownership, franchisement, patriarchal gender norms, whiteness, and more, which have served to organize members of society by extending abilities to some and generating dis-abilities for others, limiting (and sometimes destroying) peoples' capacity for movement, their ability to access resources, and their social, economic, and political power.

Juxtaposing race/racism and disability/ableism allows a confrontation of terms and social systems that is historically and politically situated. With this method, we can anchor both theory and practice in our ongoing, dynamic social world.

Conclusion

There is a deep sense in which race and disability have always worked in tandem, relying on one another to produce categories of people that can be marginalized, exploited, and made expendable, conceptually justifying violent actions by the state. In this way, "race" and "disability" are signifiers that are continually molded and formed, oftentimes by dominant powers, but also in manners resistant to state manipulation. Disability justice demands building conceptions of disability that work against the grain of dominant ways of knowing and acting. It requires an emphasis on the instability of the category of disability, especially as it relates to ongoing histories of racialized violence, and the need to identify the *un*naturalness of many experiences of disability (even, and perhaps especially, as they may not be categorized as "disability"). Resistance here involves both the critical *dismantling* of dominant political maneuverings of race and disability by state actors, institutions, and interpersonal patterns of relating and the critical *construction* of new ways of knowing, acting, relating, and redistributing resources.

Key to analyzing some of the examples discussed in this chapter is understanding racialization and disablement *in tandem* with and *reliant on* one another. Consider again the case of Flint, Michigan. Here, primarily Black and Brown folks were used for purposes of financial expediency. By drawing on a history of racialization that continues to dis-able people of color by placing them within the realm of sub-humanity and as second-class citizens who are *expected* to suffer and thereby become expendable, state and bureaucratic mechanisms of power further debilitated and disabled residents of Flint. In the even more recent example of COVID-19 mitigation practices, the fact that Black and Brown folks were undergoing higher rates of transmission, disease, and death was not used to bolster prevention but to *lessen* it since these populations were already *expected* to suffer unevenly *and* to be scapegoated in the matter of their own suffering.

This discussion of racialized disablement is meant to show that one cannot analyze present-day dynamics through singular axes of identity or oppression, isolated temporal moments, or without attention to sociopolitical contexts. We must understand the chronicity of injustice as accumulating and compounding harm via both exceptional and mundane violence that is generated by the state, institutions, and dominant social mores. Uncovering this simultaneous temporality is key to understanding the precise nature of harm inflicted on marginalized communities and how it persists.

In acknowledging the widespread nature of the sociopolitical production of disability, new conceptual tools are required to help illuminate and prevent this phenomenon. Racialized disablement is one attempt to name the specific intersection of processes of racialization and disablement. This vocabulary can be used in the context of law to motivate claims for reparation for racialized people. It can also be used in the field of healthcare and medicine as a pedagogical tool for understanding the depths to which the historical intertwinement of race and disability impact health inequities today and to prevent simplistic cultural or genetic understandings of health inequities. Above all, we must denaturalize disability as inhering in individual bodies and shift focus to the conditions of disability's emergence, which is so often tied to contexts of ongoing structural oppression. In so doing, we can attend to the alleviation of such structural patterns of violence, a task most pressing and essential to projects of racial and disability justice.

Notes

1 For more on this racial value gap, see Eddie S. Glaude Jr. (2016).
2 For a more thorough and nuanced discussion of white supremacy and abled normativity, see Joel M. Reynolds (2022).
3 My use of (racialized) "disablement" incorporates Jasbir Puar's rendering of debilitation as the "slow wearing down of populations." However, whereas Puar argues for the use of "debilitation" over disablement to name the "racialization of bodies that are expected to endure pain, suffering, and injury" and to capture disability experiences often not recognized as such, I use the term disablement here to force a conceptual reckoning between "race" and "disability." Though there is a rich literature identifying historical instances of disability being used to justify forms of white supremacy, anti-immigrant sentiment, and impoverishment, conceptual analysis of race and of disability has remained fairly distinct. I therefore juxtapose these terms in the phrase "racialized disablement" to help build a better understanding of the present interplay of healthcare systems, policing procedures, economic organization, and societal valuation schemas that produce disablement that is racialized and classes of racialized people that are dis-ableized or made to experience the world in a dis-abling way.
4 In focusing on the sociopolitical processes generating what we come to know as "race" and "disability," I am not suggesting a wholesale rejection of identity or aiming to move away from the body and the physical. And I am also not advocating a turn to "damage-centered research" that uses ableist representations of disability (as lack, failure, deficit, etc.) to define a community singularly through its relation to pathologization. Rather, we need to foreground how literal, material, physical experiences come to be, how processes of racialization and disablement *materialize* bodies— bodies that are then categorized, enumerated, responded to but also themselves respond. In this sense, racialized disablement is a term meant to empower one conceptually, a term to both call out and to claim and ultimately one to invoke hesitation at the impulse to demarcate race and disability as separate, discrete, phenomena.

Work Cited

Avril Minich, Julie. 2016. "Enabling Whom? Critical Disability Studies Now," *Lateral* 5 (1).
Bassett, Mary T. and Sandro Galeo. 2020. "Reparations as a Public Health Priority—A Strategy for Ending Black-White Health Disparities." *The New England Journal of Medicine* 383 (22): 2101–2103.
Baynton, Douglas C. 2016. *Defectives in the Land: Disability and Immigration in the Age of Eugenics*. Chicago: The University of Chicago Press.
Beesley, Kristen. 2020. "The Twin Pandemics of Racism and COVID-19." *Psychology Today*, June 16, 2020. https://www.psychologytoday.com/us/blog/psychoanalysis-unplugged/202006/the-twin-pandemics-racism-and-covid-19
Chapman, Audrey R. 2022. "Rethinking the Issue of Reparations for Black Americans." *Bioethics* 36 (3): 235–242.

Chirindo, Kundai, Robert Gutierrez-Perez, Matthew Houdek, Louis M. Maraj, Ersula J. Ore, Kendall R. Phillips, Lee M. Pierce, and G. Mitchell Reyes. 2020. "Coda: A Rupture in Time." *Women's Studies in Communication* 43 (4): 459–470.

Cooper Owens, Deirdre. 2017. *Medical Bondage: Race, Gender, and the Origins of American Gynecology.* Athens: University of Georgia Press.

COVID-19 Working Group of New York. 2020. "Chronic Injustice: Centering Equitable Health Care and Policies for COVID-19 and Other Chronic Conditions." March 2020: 3. https://nblch.org/wp-content/uploads/2021/03/Chronice_Injustice_report_March_2021.pdf

Crawford-Roberts, Ann, Sonya Shadravan, Jennifer Tsai, Nicolás E. Barceló, Allie Gips, Michael Mensah, Nichole Roxas, Alina Kung, Anna Darby, Naya Misa, Isabella Morton, Alice Shen. 2020. "George Floyd's Autopsy and the Structural Gaslighting of America." *Scientific American*, June 6, 2020. https://blogs.scientificamerican.com/voices/george-floyds-autopsy-and-the-structural-gaslighting-of-america/

Dilts, Andrew. 2012. "Incurable Blackness: Criminal Disenfranchisement, Mental Disability, and the White Citizen." *Disability Studies Quarterly* 32 (3). https://dsq-sds.org/index.php/dsq/article/view/3268/3101

Du Bois, W.E.B. 1920. *Darkwater: Voices from within the Veil.* New York: Harcourt, Brace, and Howe.

Elingon, John. 2020. "Black Doctor Dies of COVID-19 After Complaining of Racist Treatment." *New York Times*, December 23, 2020. https://www.nytimes.com/2020/12/23/us/susan-moore-black-doctor-indiana.html

Erevelles, Nirmalla. 2011. *Disability and Difference in Global Contexts: Enabling a Transformative Body Politic.* New York: Palgrave MacMillan.

Erevelles, Nirmalla. 2019. "'Scenes of Subjection' in Public Education: Thinking Intersectionally as If Disability Matters." *Educational Studies* 55 (6): 592–605.

Estes, Nick. 2019. *Our History is the Future: Standing Rock Versus the Dakota Access Pipeline, and the Long Tradition of Indigenous Resistance.* New York: Verso.

Reuters. 2020. "Fact check: 94% of individuals with additional causes of death still had COVID-19," *Reuters*, September 3, 2020. https://www.reuters.com/article/uk-factcheck-94-percent-covid-among-caus/fact-check-94-of-individuals-with-additional-causes-of-death-still-had-covid-19-idUSKBN25U2IO.

Gary, Mercer. 2021. "Disability and Debility under Neoliberal Globalization." *Feminist Studies* 47 (3): 683–699.

Gorman, Rachel. 2016. "Disablement in and For Itself: Towards a "Global" Idea of Disability." *Somatechnics* 6 (2): 249–261.

Hamilton, Darrick, William Darity Jr., Anne E. Price, Vishnu Sridharan, Rebecca Tippett. 2015. "Umbrellas Don't Make It Rain: Why Studying and Working Hard Isn't Enough for Black Americans." *The National Asset Scorecard and Communities of Color (NASCC).* http://insightcced.org/wp-content/uploads/2015/08/Umbrellas_Dont_Make_It_Rain_Final.pdf

Hartman, Saidiya. 2020. "The End of White Supremacy, An American Romance." *BOMB Magazine*, June 5, 2020. https://bombmagazine.org/articles/2020/06/05/the-end-of-white-supremacy-an-american-romance/

Jampel, Catherine. 2018. "Intersections of Disability Justice, Racial Justice, and Environmental Justice." *Environmental Sociology* 4 (1): 122–135.

Jampel, Catherine and Anthony Bebbington. 2018. "Disability Studies and Developmental Geography: Empirical Connections, Theoretical Resonances, and Future Directions." *Geography Compass* 12 (12): e12414. https://doi.org/10.1111/gec3.12414

Kang, Miliann. 2010. *The Managed Hand.* Berkeley: University of California Press.

Kim, Jina B. 2017. "Toward a Crip-of-Color Critique." *Lateral* 6 (1). https://csalateral.org/issue/6-1/forum-alt-humanities-critical-disability-studies-crip-of-color-critique-kim/

McCarty, Brett. 2020. "Moral Moments in Medicine." *The Kenan Institute of Ethics at Duke University*, November 12, 2020. https://kenan.ethics.duke.edu/moral-moments-in-medicine/

McNicholas, Celine and Margaret Poydock. 2020. "Who are essential workers? A comprehensive look at their wages, demographics, and unionization rates." *Economic Policy Institute: Working Economics Blog*, May 19, 2020. https://www.epi.org/blog/who-are-essential-workers-a-comprehensive-look-at-their-wages-demographics-and-unionization-rates/

McRuer, Robert. 2018. *Crip Times: Disability, Globalization, and Resistance.* New York: New York University Press.

Moore, Leroy and Lisa Gray-Garcia. 2020. "Disability Rights Activists Take on Twin Pandemics of Racist Police Brutality & COVID-19." *Democracy Now!*, July 13, 2020. https://www.democracynow.org/2020/7/13/disability_rights_activists_take_on_twin

National Academy of Medicine. 2020. "Medical Education and the Twin Pandemics: COVID 19 and Structural Racism." National Academy of Medicine. https://nam.edu/event/medical-education-and-the-twin-pandemics-covid-19-and-structural-racism-interest-group-09-2020-annual-meeting/

Nir, Sarah Maslin. 2015a. "The Price of Nice Nails." *The New York Times*, May 7, 2015. https://www.nytimes.com/2015/05/10/nyregion/at-nail-salons-in-nyc-manicurists-are-underpaid-and-unprotected.html

Nir, Sarah Maslin. 2015b. "Perfect Nails, Poisoned Workers." *The New York Times*, May 8, 2015. https://www.nytimes.com/2015/05/11/nyregion/nail-salon-workers-in-nyc-face-hazardous-chemicals.html

Oliver, Michael. 1990. *The Politics of Disablement: A Sociological Approach*. London: Palgrave.

Oliver, Michael and Colin Barnes. 2012. *The New Politics of Disablement*. New York: Palgrave Macmillan.

Puar, Jasbir. 2017. *The Right to Maim: Debility, Capacity, Disability*. Durham: Duke University Press.

Pulrang, Andrew. 2021. "What Disabled People Are Thinking and Feeling About the Pandemic, One Year Later." *Forbes*, May 21, 2021. https://www.forbes.com/sites/andrewpulrang/2021/03/21/what-disabled-people-are-thinking-and-feeling-about-the-pandemic-one-year-later/?sh=33ca9bc33277

Reynolds, Joel M. 2022. "Disability and White Supremacy." *Critical Philosophy of Race* 10 (1): 48–70.

Ribet, Beth. 2011. "Emergent Disability and the Limits of Equality: A Critical Reading of the UN Convention on the Rights of Persons with Disabilities." *Yale Human Rights and Development Law Journal* 14 (1): 155–204.

Roberts, Dorothy E. 1999. *Killing the Black Body: Race, Reproduction, and the Meaning of Liberty*. New York: Random House.

Russell, Marta. 2002. *Beyond Ramps: Disability at the End of the Social Contract*. Monroe, ME: Common Courage Press.

Russell, Marta. 2019. *Capitalism and Disability: Selected Writings*. Chicago: Haymarket Books.

Russell, Marta and Jean Stewart. 2001. "Disablement, Prison, and Historical Segregation." *Monthly Review: An Independent Socialist Magazine*, July 1, 2001. https://monthlyreview.org/2001/07/01/disablement-prison-and-historical-segregation/

Santa Clara University. 2020. "Twin Pandemics Forum Addresses COVID-19 and Racial Injustice." *Santa Clara University*, September 24, 2020. https://www.scu.edu/news-and-events/press-releases/2020/september-2020/twin-pandemics-forum-addresses-covid-19-and-racial-injustice.html

Schalk, Sami. 2017. "Critical Disability Studies as Methodology." *Lateral* 6 (1). https://csalateral.org/issue/6-1/forum-alt-humanities-critical-disability-studies-methodology-schalk/

Schweik, Susan M. 2009. *The Ugly Laws: Disability in Public*. New York: New York University Press.

Skinner-Dorkeno, Allison L., Apoorva Sarmal, Kashina G. Rogbeer, Chloe G. André, Bhumi Patel, Leah Cha. 2022. "Highlighting COVID-19 Racial Disparities Can Reduce Support for Safety Precautions among White U.S. Residents." *Social Science and Medicine* 301: 114951. https://doi.org/10.1016/j.socscimed.2022.114951

Silverstein, Jason. 2019. "The Healthcare Case for Reparations." *Vice News*, June 19, 2019. https://www.vice.com/en/article/5973yq/the-healthcare-case-for-reparations-hr40

Soled, Derek Ross, Avik Chatterjee, Daniele Olveczky, and Edwin G. Lindo. 2021. "The Case for Health Reparations." *Frontiers in Public Health* 9. https://doi.org/10.3389/fpubh.2021.664783

Sullivan, Shannon. 2013. "Inheriting Racist Disparities in Health: Epigenetics and the Transgenerational Effects of White Racism." *Critical Philosophy of Race* 1 (2): 190–218.

Levin, Bess. 2022. "Louisiana Senator Bill Cassidy: Our Maternal Death Rates are Only Bad if You Count Black Women." *Vanity Fair*, May 20, 2022. https://www.vanityfair.com/news/2022/05/bill-cassidy-maternal-mortality-rates.

Táíwò, Olúfẹ́mi O. 2022. *Reconsidering Reparations*. Oxford: Oxford University Press.

Tuck, Eve. 2009. "Suspending Damage: A Letter to Communities." *Harvard Educational Review* 79 (3): 409–427.

Walcott, Rinaldo. 2020. "Nothing New Here to See: How COVID-19 and State Violence Converge on Black Life." *TOPIA: Canadian Journal of Cultural Studies* 41: 158–163.

Washington, Harriet A. 2006. *Medical Apartheid: The Dark History of Medical Experimentation on Black Americans from Colonial Times to Present*. New York: Random House.

Weheliye, Alexander G. 2014. *Habeas Viscus: Racializing Assemblages, Biopolitics, and Black Feminist Theories of the Human*. Durham: Duke University Press.

Yancy, George. 2023. "Ableism Enables All Forms of Inequity and Hampers All Liberation Efforts," *Truthout*, January 3, 2023. https://truthout.org/articles/ableism-enables-all-forms-of-inequity-and-hampers-all-liberation-efforts/

6

LONG COVID AND DISABILITY

Navigating the Future

Nicholas G. Evans

Long COVID is a name given to a large cluster of continuing symptoms that can persist months, or years, after contracting coronavirus disease 2019 (Alwan 2021; Callard and Perego 2021, hereafter I use "COVID" as my acronym, rather than "COVID-19" etc). Much remains unknown about long COVID, but what we do know is that in its severe manifestations it can compromise an individual's ability to live—at least in our world—a good life. Individuals suffering long COVID may report fatigue, cognitive symptoms such as difficulty concentrating and impaired memory, and sensory changes like permanent loss of smell or taste (Hampshire et al. 2021). Physiologically, long COVID may cause damage to extremities, in some cases requiring amputation (Lee et al. 2022; Alattar et al. 2021); multiorgan injury such as chronic kidney disease requiring dialysis or transplant (Iacobucci 2020; Yende and Parikh 2021); or respiratory complications and persistent post-exertional symptoms. These symptoms may exist in isolation or in clusters, and though they range in severity, many greatly affect people's wellbeing and life plans. Long COVID may have visible symptoms (e.g. so-called "COVID-toes," arising from damage to extremities through loss of circulation), but most are frequently invisible to others (Hereth et al. 2022).

The idea of persistent symptoms arising from infections is not novel. The most obvious cases are those in which the virus continues to replicate in a human host over an extended period. HIV is a clear, though often exceptional case (Benton 2015) owing to the mechanics of lentiviruses and their ability to remain protected in host tissue. The sustained replication of diseases such as Ebola virus disease in immunologically privileged sites in the body such as the eye (Shantha, Crozier, and Yeh 2017) constitutes a persistent disease; as does the extensive period, confirmed only in 2017, in which the Ebola virus can remain latent in human seminal fluid. Besides these, however, it is possible to experience sustained symptoms arising from immunological responses to viruses including influenza, other SARS-like viruses, Zika virus, and dengue; malaria and lyme diseases, caused by parasites; and e. coli, anthrax, botulism, gangrene, and other bacterial infections. We've known about these "post-infection sequelae" arguably as long as we've known about the microbiological basis for disease: the 1918 influenza pandemic saw the rise of "encephalitis lethargica" (Hoffman and Vilensky 2017), a cousin to long COVID. Perhaps by way of analogy, a condition resembling long COVID in

DOI: 10.4324/9781003502623-9

much the same way "shell shock" resembled, and later came to be replaced by post-traumatic stress disorder, in the way that invisible, marginalized (and *marginalizing*) impairments can be "discovered" more than once.

These long-term post-viral syndromes can be extremely impairing to an individual's life and wellbeing. Their neurocognitive versions, moreover, can compromise an individuals' long-term prospects in a modern social order that places overwhelming emphasis on non-stop activity and is exceedingly demanding of executive function. This makes syndromes like long COVID, on their face, good candidates for being understood as *disabilities*. That is, they are— depending on how one understands what constitutes a disability—either long-term physiological conditions that undermine an individual's wellbeing, or differences that form the basis of marginalization, or both (Evans, Reynolds, and Johnson 2021).

In August 2022 I and some colleagues made the case that long COVID constituted a disability and that it posed serious challenges for policy (Hereth et al. 2022). In this chapter, I want to recanvas these ideas with an additional two years of insight into long COVID, its trajectory, and the voices that arose around the condition. In the interests of space and given the conceptual depth of this volume, I will not spend too much time rehearsing the long-standing debate between welfarist, medical, social, and other conceptions of disability. Rather, I will proceed as follows. First, I will outline a series of *pro tanto* reasons to understand long COVID as a disability *in some sense*, and a series of nuances to understanding long COVID as such. Second, I will talk about the politics of the moment in which we find ourselves, recognizing post-infection sequelae as disabilities. Third, I will talk about what long COVID might tell us about disability rights, disability justice, and what understanding long COVID as a disability means for thinking about future pandemics, climate change, and other emerging crises.

Disability

Long COVID is disabling. I will not spend extensive amounts of time on whether, for example, disability is better understood as "mere difference" or "bad difference." This is because, from qualitative work on long COVID, the syndrome is a kind of intersection between these two categories: one in which, there are strong reasons to understand the causal relation between difference and welfare both as a bad difference, and as a mere difference. Long COVID is miserable for many; but it's also often, particularly in its neurocognitive manifestations, a difference that I suspect in other social arrangements would not be nearly as impairing as it is today (Callard and Perego 2021).

What makes long COVID interesting, I believe, are the following properties. In many cases, long COVID mirrors the experiences of communities who have previously fought long, terrible fights to be recognized as disabled and receive understanding, attention, and accommodation as a result. What is remarkable about long COVID is the speed with which it was initially recognized, but also the way that interest in the condition has waxed and waned society-wide along the same rhythms of the "panic and neglect" cycle of infectious diseases themselves.

Consider the resemblance between long COVID and myalgic encephalomyelitis/chronic fatigue syndrome (ME/CFS) in terms of its symptomatology. ME/CFS was first diagnosed as early as 1934 in terms that are extremely like our modern understanding of it, but it later came to be subsumed into theories of hysteria in 1970s psychiatry: the condition had the prefix "benign" that was only dropped in 1986. Fast forward to the last twenty years and ME/CFS has been increasingly recognized as a post-viral syndrome, though debate remains about through which viruses, and what mechanism, the syndrome is triggered (Hanson 2023). This kind of century-long struggle to recognition, among others, has surely motivated the urgency of recognizing long COVID as, if not a disability, something to invest resources and attention into.

This doesn't mean, however, that the properties that make long COVID disabling are unique to long COVID. Rather—as I'll discuss in the next section—long COVID has emerged in a way that sheds light on a series of properties about disabilities that are, I think, less appreciated in the literature on long COVID than they should be. Importantly, this has implications for our understanding of disability.

First, long COVID is an *acquired* disability. That is, whereas many disability theorists utilize congenital syndromes as their paradigms (Barnes 2016), long COVID has a causal, temporal relation to a person's identity and life plan. If we understand long COVID to be a disability, those who experience it do so with an idea of "before long COVID" and "having long COVID." Moreover, the causal relation between one's impairment and government inaction, or neglect, is palpable in the case of long COVID, meaning that long COVID is not merely acquired but frequently has been *imposed* on those who experience it (This is related to scholarship on "debility," e.g. Puar 2017; Erevelles 2011). Much as we tend to capture war in terms of deaths and not disability, we might imagine that the social murder (to borrow a term from Engels) of COVID, expressed only in deaths, obscures the wider harm of our social institutions in the face of pandemic disease.

Second, long COVID is, for many though not all, a *transient* disability. That is, there is a before long COVID, a having long COVID, and a third "after long COVID." What makes long COVID particularly interesting, however, is the extreme variation in how long someone might exist as disabled—or, as I'll talk about a little later, acutely disabled. In the UK, the Coronavirus Infection Survey conducted from April 2020 to August 2021 estimated that between 3% and 11% of 15,061 participants with COVID infection experienced symptoms for more than 12 weeks (Office for National Statistics 2021). The US Centers for Disease Control and Prevention (Bull-Otterson 2022) found up to 20% of 353,000 patients aged 18–64 years had one symptom attributable to COVID more than four weeks after infection. Depending on your definition, you can have long COVID for 1–3 months as the *de minimus* criteria on which the syndrome is understood, *or* you can have it if not permanently (the pandemic has only existed for four years), then at least indefinitely. However, given the homology between long COVID and ME/CFS, it is not unreasonable to expect that there will be an extremely wide range of timeframes over which the former can occur, and for some it will be permanent.

Third, long COVID is for most an *invisible* disability. It does not have any essential physical signifiers that act to inform others that one is disabled, whether at the level of one's body (e.g. an amputation) or a common assistive device (e.g. a cane). Individuals with invisible disabilities find it more difficult to find recognition among their families, the public, medical practitioners, and the law (N. A. Davis 2005). Individuals with long COVID may also struggle to self-identify as disabled in cases where their preconceptions of what it means to be disabled are suddenly confronted with their new lived experience, as reported last year:

Long COVID is often imperceptible in casual interactions, which forces long-haulers to contend with disclosure and the possibility of passing as able-bodied. One such long-hauler is Julia Moore Vogel, a program director at Scripps Research, who initially hesitated at the idea of getting a disabled-parking permit. "My first thought was, I'm not disabled, because I can walk," she told me. But if she did walk, she'd be drained for days. Taking her daughter to the zoo or the beach was out of the question.

(Ryan 2023)

Fourth, and related to the above, long COVID is a disability around which a community has formed for activism, but one largely targeting treatment and cure (Callard and Perego 2021). People with long COVID often *self-identify as ill* and *wish to be cured*. This points to one of the key strategies that some individuals have adopted in recognizing themselves and their community as disabled: to mobilize medical and political power toward their recognition and to an end to their suffering. In this case, it is often toward greater emphasis on diagnosis, treatment, and cure, and it has been explicitly connected to the struggle for HIV/AIDS treatments in the 1980s given its tactics and goals (Curwen 2021).

This makes individuals with long COVID disabled in a contested and very particular sense. Individuals may be disabled through long COVID, the harm caused by their symptoms, its relation to our social framework, or both. Those effects can be severe: one international survey in 2020 of 3,762 people in 56 countries with confirmed or suspected COVID who had illness lasting over 28 days found that 45% of respondents had required a reduced work schedule and another 23% had left the workforce because of suspected long COVID (H. E. Davis et al. 2021). Long COVID in children and young people could similarly jeopardize educational attainment. However, individuals with long COVID may not understand their impairments as permanent; nor as a part of their identity internally or as they present to the world; and they may not even regard themselves as disabled at all. If they do understand themselves as disabled, qualitative data to date suggests that they do so in a way that is focused on their pursuit of recognition, treatment, and cure. One upshot of this is that individuals with long COVID, if they do understand themselves to be disabled, may not understand themselves—or be understood by others—to be part of a community of disability formed around a shared identity, but instead, in their case, around the discrete event of the pandemic.

Recognition

This sense in which long COVID is a distinct form of disability has two important implications. The first of these implications has to do with long COVID's capacity to be recognized socially and politically as a disability, and whether such recognition serves the long COVID community *per se*, as they appear to understand their interests.

On the one hand, it appears that long COVID does not necessarily need recognition for already having it. The US National Institutes of Health (NIH), at the time of writing, has to date invested more than a billion dollars in long COVID research. However, it is important to understand these numbers in the context of government medical research: this places long COVID in about the same ballpark as epilepsy research, a bit more than traumatic brain injury research, and a little less than schizophrenia. It pales in comparison to the US $3 billion HIV/AIDS *annual* earmark, for example. Nonetheless, when compared to other disabilities, and given that long COVID is only four years old, this is an astonishing win for that community.

However, long COVID is likely, I suspect, tied to larger forces that mediate societal responses to pandemic disease. The fortunes of long COVID research funding might, for example, only persist so long as the government continues to support the idea that COVID is a threat and is a threat that is the proper province of government action. I suspect, however, that this will change rapidly over the coming few years as new challenges supplant the current foci of government voices and priorities.

Most recent coverage has borne this out. For all its investment, the NIH has been characteristically slow to respond to long COVID with clinical trials, investigational therapy, or even the sharing of results from ongoing observational studies (Ladyzhets and Zhang 2023). We might then expect the long COVID community to continue to push for additional funding and action, noting the frequency with which the syndrome emerges under conditions of repeat infection and its ongoing prevalence. The politics of recognition of disease are rife with contested metaphors and performative strategies.

It appears that there are two ways to go in this vein. The first would be to double down on long COVID qua *disease*. In particular, the fatigue-inducing aspects of long COVID might represent a threat to long-term productivity of the nation, in the way that Alzheimer's or obesity (which, while distinctly not a disease, is *characterized as such*) are taken to represent profound economic drains and even threats to national security (Popkin 2011). That is, we might expect long COVID to be framed as a threat to national security because of its neurocognitive and productivity costs.

The other would be to double down on long COVID qua *disability*. That is, rather than the punitive exercise of power that often accompanies the securitization of disease (Evans 2023), we might say that as a disability, individuals with long COVID deserve substantial supports for their lives independent of an alleviation of their symptoms. The reasons for this are threefold. First, there is a simple intrinsic value to supporting individuals with poor health states, which can be tied among other things to the self-respect of citizens: our social contract is, and should be, designed on the idea that each citizen's expectations to pursue their life plans should be protected continuous with those of others. Framed this way, long COVID—and other post-infection syndromes—are an expected disruption to our life plans, ought to be guarded against where possible, and ought to receive support when needed.

The second is that even small disruptions in the capacity of individuals to participate in social life can be devastating absent a society-wide framework within which to receive support. Recall that a significant proportion of individuals with long COVID leave the workplace, even if only temporarily. We know, however, that even short departures from work can differentially affect individuals, and their descendants, in their ability to carry out their life plans through lost earnings and opportunities. Long COVID is thus "dysgenic": it marginalizes a large class of people across society (Evans, Reynolds, and Johnson 2021). Reducing this is, again, something in everyone's interests, as the costs of supporting individuals who suffer from this form of marginalization will undoubtedly fall to marginalized people themselves, who form the bulk of unpaid and unsupported care work worldwide (Moehler 2017).

The third is that individuals with at least some types of non-long COVID disabilities are more likely to end up with long COVID and suffer from its more severe effects (Subramanian et al. 2022). There is thus a reason for the *disability community* itself to enter a fight for long COVID. That is, the recognition of long COVID as a disability is not just solidarity borne of the effects that individuals with other disabilities can relate to, but one of self-preservation. At least as far as surviving what might be now called the "chronic" (as opposed to acute) stage of the pandemic, increasing resources to counteract the worst of long COVID's symptoms—as well as putting in place a social welfare system that supports individuals who do end up with those symptoms—is aligns with core interests of the disability community writ large.

But herein, I suspect, lies the rub. On the one hand, it is well understood that some individuals with disabilities can have trouble accessing the disability community because they cannot recognize themselves as such or because they struggle to be recognized as disabled by the disability community (Shakespeare, Ndagire, and Seketi 2021). So, it is not as simple as saying that people with long COVID and people with non-long COVID disabilities ought to support one another. Recognition goes both ways, and one of the striking things about the disability literature during the pandemic is the way it has largely *not* addressed long COVID. For example, a special issue of *Disability Studies Quarterly* on COVID containing an incredible geographic and conceptual scope mentions "long haulers" in its opening editorial (Block et al. 2021), but only engaged long COVID once and only in passing (Rodriguez 2021).

This shouldn't, however, be taken as a mark against the disability community. As a 2021 issue of the Disability Rights Monitor concluded, many of the effects of the pandemic *response* were worse than the pandemic itself. That community was in crisis response to everything from scarce resource allocation paradigms (Sabatello et al. 2020) to homelessness and unemployment that disproportionately affected people with disabilities (Evans 2023, chapter 2) to keeping personal ventilators from being reallocated upon entry to the ICU (Reynolds, Guidry-Grimes, and Savin 2021) to the high-level dismissal of vulnerable populations as "falling by the wayside" in justifying relaxed approaches to later waves of the pandemic (Phillips 2023).

Is there a reason to suspect that this lack of recognition might ultimately become entrenched? I suspect so. Recall the sudden investment in scientific research to understand and address long COVID—a mobilization of resources that is significantly more than most disabilities. I suspect this is, or will be, seen as fundamentally unfair by some segments of the heterogenous and diverse disability community. That is, if you are someone with ME/CFS, or RSD, or any number of other disabilities that are increasingly connected to post-infection sequelae, you might see long COVID sufferers as extracting resources at a speed that is decades faster than your disease took to be recognized *as a disease*. This is a spot where envy might emerge. By envy, however, I don't mean the mere emotion, but rather the phenomenon that arises when rational, otherwise reasonable actors look upon the gains of others within our social framework as a kind of loss for themselves (Rawls 2009, esp. ch.4).

Two things need to be reinforced here. One is that this envy is unlikely to be homogenous and may also be temporally fixed depending upon how the story of long COVID continues to play out. In 2022, a Washington Post article entitled, "How long COVID could change the way we think about disability," articulated this point clearly; Diana Zicklin Berrent, who founded the long-COVID group Survivor Corps, noted that there were resentments from other disability activists, for whom the feeling described was "we've been out here screaming from the rooftops for decades, and you guys show up." This, however, speaks to the rationality of this kind of position. given the history of neglect of disabilities writ large, but also the deep histories of individual disabilities, it may be rational to view the gains of the long-COVID community as a form of unfairness, or at least meet them with skepticism. Scientific resources are scarce. Scarcer than they should be, as ultimately the state underfunds science and medicine as connected to the primary goods of citizens, but still scarce: there are only so many dollars and scientists to go around for the sheer variety of biomedical problems out there, even just those that have direct material implications for individuals. For a group to suddenly matter at the level of policy, particularly when they suffer from a condition that is alike many others, may on some level be seen as an injustice. This can be seen within individual disease types, for example, in the way that activism around HIV/AIDS has historically excluded the voices of women, non-whites (and non-American people of color in particular), incarcerated individuals, and other groups that bear the disproportionate burden of HIV/AIDS but have received the smallest representative share of resources for treatment and prevention (Diallo 2021; Morabia 2021; Amaro and Prado 2021; Beletsky et al. 2021).

Refusal by the long COVID community to identify with, or ally themselves with individuals who share these challenges, may also be seen as a form of ableism. Tom Shakespeare, among others, has addressed the othering that arises when individuals don't recognize themselves as "disabled" due to fears about what understanding themselves as such entails (Shakespeare 1999). At the level of a group decision, intentional or not, there is likely a performative at play that on the one hand secures resources but at the same time does not engage in recognition of others with similar interests. "We are not defined by our disease." This, despite the acknowledgement that ME/CFS and long COVID are likely similar, if not the same biological mechanism of disease, and both are among a larger family of impairments that cause suffering and marginalization.

The politics of recognition is an ancient problem: what happens when a new group enters our public sphere that speaks for, speaks over, or ignores a pre-existing group? Long COVID features in high profile arenas such as the *BMJ, Nature, New York Times, STAT*, and even *Buzzfeed* abound with articles describing how individuals with long COVID may find their symptoms dismissed, ignored or downplayed: but these pieces do nothing to connect long COVID to disability (instead comparing this experience to those with "chronic illness," as well as women, people of color, and fat people).

The use of "chronic illness" in these cases is instructive: even when it's *right there*, many ignore the D-word.

What comes of this will surely shape the politics of infectious disease and disability alike for years to come. Recognizing post-infection sequelae as an expected part of infectious disease, as I'll detail in the next section, changes our understanding of the threat of infectious disease. But, to paraphrase Katie Eyer (2021), "what does 'nothing about us without us' mean when the 'us' expands?"

Futures

There is a tension, then, between the marked rise in disability in the world through long COVID—recognized, or otherwise—and what this means for disability culture and politics. But I think this is resolvable. Here is a strategy for reform and for more radical change.

The reform piece is quite simple. Pandemic preparedness that does not start from a critical understanding of disability is inequitable by design. Pandemics cause disability; pandemics prey on disability. And government inaction, negligence, or malfeasance deepens the marginalization, discrimination, and disadvantage that arises from being disabled in an ableist world.

Consider a military analogy. We frequently report deaths from armed conflict, but not injuries. Particularly among civilian casualties, this often means the full scope of war is vastly underreported. A precise measure is extremely difficult to attain due to the conditions of armed conflict itself, but in the last decade of the twentieth century, it ranged from nine to *thirty-three* years of life negatively impacted by injury and disability—in disability-adjusted life years—to every 1 year lost to combat *death* (Murray 2002).[1] We think of "mass casualty events" as mass *death* events, but death is the tip of the iceberg in terms of the harms inflicted upon us.

Reframing mass casualty events as a disability issue emphasizes two things. First, it emphasizes that evaluating the outcomes of pandemics should not only encompass harm inflicted on the dead, but on the living too. The scope and scale of harms accruing to newly or historically disabled people—imperfect as our measures are—is vast, even in comparison to death. And this scope and scale has multiple senses. As evinced by long COVID, contracting an infectious disease can be a disabling event, for which our society is ill-equipped to support at the best of times but especially under the resource constraints brought about by decades of neglect for appropriate pandemic preparedness, failures for which governments are liable (Nicholas G. Evans 2023, chapters 9 and 10). The misdeeds of pandemic response, moreover, derail lives and harm individuals through the arrangement of our social conditions *even if one doesn't contract* a pandemic infectious disease. Finally, these former kinds of harm accrue disproportionately to individuals with disabilities who are more likely to contract long COVID; are more likely to be the victims of the social murder of the pandemic response; and are more likely to be harmed multiple times over in terms of the disproportionate association between disability and poverty, disability and negative racialization, disability and gender differences, and so on.

As above, the individuals most likely to experience long COVID include the disabled, among other marginalized groups. It is no secret that COVID's outcomes track widespread patterns of marginalization (Johnson and Martin 2020). But as long COVID amply demonstrated, pandemics also *create* new forms of marginalization and their attendant harms.

Second, support for the survivors of pandemics can draw from the wisdom of the disability community (see Sarah Miller's chapter in this volume). Because long COVID is not a monolith, the kinds of support those who experience it will require are often accessibility and accommodation support we should already expect—and provide—for those with relevant disabilities. Executive and cognitive impairments, mobility disorders, chronic pain, and more are staples of many sorts of disabilities, and best practices do exist for these even if they are rarely used. This can and should form the basis for further pandemic preparedness literature and policy which, to my knowledge, has not dealt with disability as a sustained area of focus. Larry Gostin's *Global Health Security: A Blueprint for the Future*, for example, only mentions disability in terms of "disability-adjusted life years" and the *cost* of disability to national healthcare (Gostin 2021). *Lessons from the COVID War (2023)*, whose author team includes bioethicists Ezekiel Emanuel and Ruth Faden, only mentions disability as an argument *against* virtual schooling during pandemics. While criticisms of the neglect of disability voices, scholarship, and policy appear in, for example, the literature on resource allocation (Ellison and Ballan 2023), there is room for a more thoroughgoing critique of what could be seen as a foundational misstep in the field.

But talk of accommodations gives way to a more radical project that aligns with disability justice. That is, not only the experiences of individuals with long COVID but *all* our experiences give rise to the idea that what the disability community has been advocating for years is not just good for them: it is sound and reasonable social policy in an age of global pandemics. Disabled individuals who found themselves marginalized socially and professionally prior to the COVID pandemic were suddenly able to work from home, interact online for a variety of reasons, and gain access to widespread curbside and delivery of a huge range of needs and interests. Many countries were able to provide financial support for individuals that was not means tested and did not require degrading or overburdened paperwork requirements. Telemedicine was, suddenly, a staple experience for us. *Much of this is what people with disabilities have asked for, and needed, for decades.* What was previously unreasonable as an accommodation, to use legal parlance, was suddenly ubiquitous and even expected. This means that entities who claimed such accommodations were unreasonable or too burdensome were misled, neglectful, or lying.

A movement that unites the long COVID community with the various strands of the disability community could demand a more radical project—insisting, for instance, that radical disability politics just *is pandemic preparedness.* The unceasing "we are not ready for the next pandemic" op-eds that have lined the pages of major news websites for decades now all neglect that pandemics create disability and that preventing the harms of pandemic requires making our world more accessible—it requires listening to what disabled people and the disability justice movement have been saying for ages. COVID created a world in which people were unable to move; unable to communicate effectively; unable to engage with their communities; and unable to access their basic needs. And because COVID is not gone, what we are left with is a new avenue of social marginalization through which individuals are disabled—an ever-present infectious disease.

Given the to-date $3.7 trillion price tag of long COVID in America alone, the typical economic rationales of denying accessibility seem laughable. What will be required is for individuals living with long COVID to engage in solidaristic work with the disability activists that have spent decades carving out legal and policy challenges for their communities. Not just to advance the science of long COVID—though we should do this, and in alignment with understanding post-infection sequelae writ large—but to ensure that individuals who will undoubtedly be caught in the next pandemic are able to flourish, either by avoiding unnecessary and unjust imposition of risk by poor pandemic response, or by a society who moves on from the pandemic without attending to those who have been, and continue to be, affected by it. This will have, I believe, the intended effect of ensuring that the interests of people with long COVID, and any future long haulers, are aligned with those of other disability communities in pushing for a more just world for not only disabled people, but all people, pandemic or otherwise.

Note

1 DALYs have received compelling critique by disability scholars and activists, among others. In the interest of brevity, I won't rehearse them, but rather invoke the term in a critical sense: picking out years of life impacted by disability *in an ableist world*. Disability can be, absent ableism, not negative, that is, a mere difference or even in certain cases a good difference.

Works Cited

Alattar, Khalid Omar, Farah Noaman Subhi, Ayesha Humaid Saif Alshamsi, Nadereh Eisa, Niaz Ahmed Shaikh, Jehangir Afzal Mobushar, and Asma Al Qasmi. 2021. "COVID-19-Associated Leukocytoclastic Vasculitis Leading to Gangrene and Amputation." *IDCases* 24: e01117. https://doi.org/10.1016/j.idcr.2021.e01117

Alwan, Nisreen A. 2021. "The Road to Addressing Long COVID." *Science* 373 (6554): 491–93. https://doi.org/10.1126/science.abg7113

Amaro, Hortensia, and Guillermo Prado. 2021. "Then and Now: Historical Landscape of HIV Prevention and Treatment Inequities Among Latinas." *American Journal of Public Health* 111 (7): 1246–48. https://doi.org/10.2105/AJPH.2021.306336

Barnes, Elizabeth. 2016. *The Minority Body: A Theory of Disability*. 1st ed. Oxford, UK: Oxford University Press.

Beletsky, Leo, Meaghan Thumath, Danielle F. Haley, Gregg Gonsalves, and Ayana Jordan. 2021. "HIV's Trajectory: Biomedical Triumph, Structural Failure." *American Journal of Public Health* 111 (7): 1258–60. https://doi.org/10.2105/AJPH.2021.306354

Benton, Adia. 2015. *HIV Exceptionalism: Development through Disease in Sierra Leone*. 3rd ed. Minneapolis: University of Minnesota Press.

Block, Pamela, Pereira Anah Guedes de Mello, and Dikaios Sakellariou. 2021. "Introduction to the Special Issue: Disability and COVID-19." *Disability Studies Quarterly* 41 (3). https://doi.org/10.18061/dsq.v41i3.8440

Bull-Otterson, Lara. 2022. "Post–COVID Conditions Among Adult COVID-19 Survivors Aged 18–64 and ≥65 Years — United States, March 2020–November 2021." *MMWR. Morbidity and Mortality Weekly Report* 71. https://doi.org/10.15585/mmwr.mm7121e1

Callard, Felicity, and Elisa Perego. 2021. "How and Why Patients Made Long COVID." *Social Science & Medicine (1982)* 268 (January): 113426. https://doi.org/10.1016/j.socscimed.2020.113426

Curwen, Thomas. 2021. "'Long Haul' COVID-19 Sufferers Take a Page from AIDS/HIV Activism to Be Heard." *Los Angeles Times*, April 26, 2021, sec. California. https://www.latimes.com/california/story/2021-04-26/activists-and-advocates-find-their-voice-in-the-long-haul

Davis, Hannah E., Gina S. Assaf, Lisa McCorkell, Hannah Wei, Ryan J. Low, Yochai Re'em, Signe Redfield, Jared P. Austin, and Athena Akrami. 2021. "Characterizing Long COVID in an International Cohort: 7 Months of Symptoms and Their Impact." *EClinicalMedicine* 38 (August). https://doi.org/10.1016/j.eclinm.2021.101019

Davis, N. Ann. 2005. "Invisible Disability." *Ethics* 116 (1): 153–213. https://doi.org/10.1086/453151

Diallo, Dázon D. 2021. "The Sankofa Paradox: Why Black Women Know the HIV Epidemic Ends With 'WE.'" *American Journal of Public Health* 111 (7): 1237–39. https://doi.org/10.2105/AJPH.2021.306358

Ellison, Brooke M, and Michelle Ballan. 2023. "Not My Ventilator: How Conceptual Frameworks of Disability and the Absence of the Disabled Voice Have Shaped Healthcare Policies in the COVID-19 Pandemic and Beyond." *Global Social Policy* 23 (1): 171–75. https://doi.org/10.1177/14680181221145866

Erevelles, Nirmala. 2011. "The Color of Violence: Reflecting on Gender, Race, and Disability in Wartime." In *Feminist Disability Studies*, edited by Kim Q. Hall, 117–35. Indiana University Press.

Evans, Nicholas G. 2023. *War on All Fronts: A Theory of Health Security Justice*. Cambridge, Massachusetts: The MIT Press.

Evans, Nicholas G, Joel Michael Reynolds, and Kaylee R. Johnson. 2021. "Moving through Capacity Space: Mapping Disability and Enhancement." *Journal of Medical Ethics* 47 (11): 748–55. https://doi.org/10.1136/medethics-2019-105732

Eyer, Katie. 2021. "Claiming Disability." *Boston University Law Review* 101:547.

Gostin, Lawrence O. 2021. *Global Health Security: A Blueprint for the Future*. Harvard University Press.

Group, COVID Crisis. 2023. *Lessons from the COVID War: An Investigative Report*. New York: PublicAffairs.

Hampshire, Adam, William Trender, Samuel R. Chamberlain, Amy E. Jolly, Jon E. Grant, Fiona Patrick, Ndaba Mazibuko, et al. 2021. "Cognitive Deficits in People Who Have Recovered from COVID-19." *EClinicalMedicine* 39 (September). https://doi.org/10.1016/j.eclinm.2021.101044

Hanson, Maureen R. 2023. "The Viral Origin of Myalgic Encephalomyelitis/Chronic Fatigue Syndrome." *PLOS Pathogens* 19 (8): e1011523. https://doi.org/10.1371/journal.ppat.1011523

Hereth, Blake, Paul Tubig, Ashton Sorrels, Anna Muldoon, Kelly Hills, and Nicholas G. Evans. 2022. "Long COVID and Disability: A Brave New World." *BMJ* 378 (August): e069868. https://doi.org/10.1136/bmj-2021-069868

Hoffman, Leslie A., and Joel A. Vilensky. 2017. "Encephalitis Lethargica: 100 Years after the Epidemic." *Brain* 140 (8): 2246–51. https://doi.org/10.1093/brain/awx177

Iacobucci, Gareth. 2020. "Long COVID: Damage to Multiple Organs Presents in Young, Low Risk Patients." *BMJ* 371 (November): m4470. https://doi.org/10.1136/bmj.m4470

Ladyzhets, Betsy, Rachel Cohrs Zhang. 2023. "The NIH Has Poured $1 Billion into Long COVID Research — with Little to Show for It." *STAT* (blog). April 20, 2023. https://www.statnews.com/2023/04/20/long-covid-nih-billion/

Lee, Kathryn A., Richard S. McBride, Ranjeet Narlawar, Rebecca Myers, and George A. Antoniou. 2022. "COVID Toes: Concurrent Lower Limb Arterial and Venous Thromboembolism in a Patient with COVID-19 Pneumonitis Presenting with Foot Ischaemia." *Vascular and Endovascular Surgery* 56 (2): 201–7. https://doi.org/10.1177/15385744211045600

Johnson, Akilah, and Nina Martin. 2020. "How COVID-19 Hollowed Out a Generation of Young Black Men." *ProPublica.* December 22, 2020. https://www.propublica.org/article/how-covid-19-hollowed-out-a-generation-of-young-black-men?token=XSO7CCiM7D0udJrFYQeZnvAitR3ZT0sj

Moehler, Michael. 2017. "In Defense of a Democratic Productivist Welfare State." *European Journal of Philosophy* 25 (2): 416–39. https://doi.org/10.1111/ejop.12157

Morabia, Alfredo. 2021. "AIDS Versus COVID-19: Different Profiles, Common Causes, and Common Victims." *American Journal of Public Health* 111 (7): 1175. https://doi.org/10.2105/AJPH.2021.306362

Murray, C J L. 2002. "Armed Conflict as a Public Health Problem." *BMJ* 324 (7333): 346–49. https://doi.org/10.1136/bmj.324.7333.346

Office for National Statistics. 2021. "Updated Estimates of the Prevalence of Post-Acute Symptoms among People with Coronavirus (COVID-19) in the UK," 19.

Phillips, Aleks., "Fauci Speaks out over COVID Variant as Mask Mandates Reintroduced." 2023. Newsweek. September 1, 2023. https://www.newsweek.com/anthony-fauci-new-covid-variants-hospitalizations-mask-mandates-1823981

Popkin, Barry M. 2011. "Is The Obesity Epidemic a National Security Issue Around the Globe?" *Current Opinion in Endocrinology, Diabetes, and Obesity* 18 (5): 328–31. https://doi.org/10.1097/MED.0b013e3283471c74

Puar, Jasbir K. 2017. *The Right to Maim: Debility, Capacity, Disability.* ANIMA: Critical Race Studies Otherwise. Durham, NC: Duke University Press.

Rawls, John. 2009. *A Theory of Justice.* Harvard University Press.

Reynolds, Joel Michael, Laura Guidry-Grimes, and Katie Savin. 2021. "Against Personal Ventilator Reallocation." *Cambridge Quarterly of Healthcare Ethics: CQ: The International Journal of Healthcare Ethics Committees* 30 (2): 272–84. https://doi.org/10.1017/S0963180120000833

Rodriguez, Erika. 2021. "The Essential Work of Crip Resistance: Demanding Dignity in Spain's Pandemic Austerity." *Disability Studies Quarterly* 41 (3). https://doi.org/10.18061/dsq.v41i3.8353

Ryan, Lindsay. 2023. "Long-Haulers Are Trying to Define Themselves." *The Atlantic* (blog). April 28, 2023. https://www.theatlantic.com/health/archive/2023/04/long-covid-disability-identity-advocacy/673892/

Sabatello, Maya, Teresa Blankmeyer Burke, Katherine E. McDonald, and Paul S. Appelbaum. 2020. "Disability, Ethics, and Health Care in the COVID-19 Pandemic." *American Journal of Public Health* 110 (10): 1523–27. https://doi.org/10.2105/AJPH.2020.305837

Shakespeare, Tom. 1999. "Coming Out and Coming Home." *International Journal of Sexuality and Gender Studies* 4 (1): 39–51. https://doi.org/10.1023/A:1023202424014

Shakespeare, Tom, Florence Ndagire, and Queen E. Seketi. 2021. "Triple Jeopardy: Disabled People and the COVID-19 Pandemic." *The Lancet* 397 (10282): 1331–33. https://doi.org/10.1016/S0140-6736(21)00625-5

Shantha, Jessica G., Ian Crozier, and Steven Yeh. 2017. "An Update on Ocular Complications of Ebola Virus Disease." *Current Opinion in Ophthalmology* 28 (6): 600–606. https://doi.org/10.1097/ICU.0000000000000426

Subramanian, Anuradhaa, Krishnarajah Nirantharakumar, Sarah Hughes, Puja Myles, Tim Williams, Krishna M. Gokhale, Tom Taverner, et al. 2022. "Symptoms and Risk Factors for Long COVID in Non-Hospitalized Adults." *Nature Medicine* 28 (8): 1706–14. https://doi.org/10.1038/s41591-022-01909-w

Yende, Sachin, and Chirag R. Parikh. 2021. "Long COVID and Kidney Disease." *Nature Reviews Nephrology* 17 (12): 792–93. https://doi.org/10.1038/s41581-021-00487-3

7

PATIENT-CENTERED COMMUNICATION AND RESOURCE ALLOCATION FOR NON-SPEAKING PEOPLE DURING CRISES

Ally Peabody Smith

The ideal of patient-centered care, or care oriented around an individual's unique health needs, has become standard in clinical practice (Epstein et al. 2011; Fix et al. 2018; Reynolds 2009; Santana et al. 2018). Patient-centered care strives to make medical practices collaborative between patients, their families, and clinicians; it encourages accessibility; it focuses not exclusively on physical dimensions of health but on its social and emotional components; and it urges sensitivity to patient values, cultural norms, and individual preferences. A central aspect of patient-centered care is patient-centered communication, or communication intended to ensure patient understanding and participation in their care. Clinicians practicing patient-centered communication seek to converse in ways comprehensible to the average person, avoiding unnecessary jargon and "medicalese." Healthcare workers consider each individual patient *qua* individual with their own distinct preferences and values that impact their decision-making. This chapter will discuss the myriad ways current practices of patient-centered communication fall short for non-speaking intellectually disabled patients, particularly during health crises like the COVID-19 pandemic.

There are many types of patients who cannot self-advocate or who lack decision-making capacities, including young children, those with neurodegenerative or psychiatric diagnoses, those suffering disorders of consciousness, non-native speakers lacking a translator, and those who have been systematically oppressed in such a way that they are unable to speak for themselves in a medical context. These groups – of patients who, for one reason or another, lack the ability to advance their own medical interests – fall into two main types: for some, it's a question of their individual cognitive capacities, and for others, it's a question of relations and situations. Those with non-speaking intellectual disabilities fall into the former category. For the purposes of this chapter, my discussion will remain embedded with this type of patient, who may *also* face social and political barriers such as systemic ableism, but for whom a primary practical barrier to healthcare is the inability to communicate linguistically, which is itself a result of the nature of their disability.

Improving healthcare justice for individuals with non-speaking forms of intellectual disability is an urgent project. Healthcare disparities between non-disabled and disabled patient groups are both dire and well-documented (Diab and Johnston 2004, Ervin et al. 2014, Krahn

DOI: 10.4324/9781003502623-10

et al. 2015, Okoro et al. 2018, WHO 2016). Although there are doubtless many causes contributing to the injustices faced by those with intellectual disability, and while there has been little research conducted specifically comparing intellectually disabled to either disabled but non-intellectually disabled, or non-disabled people, it stands to reason that due to pervasive ableist beliefs about intellectual disability and because of communicative and access issues, those with intellectual disabilities are amongst the most marginalized groups (Inclusion International 2020, Peabody Smith and Feinsinger 2024). This lack of consideration is sometimes reflected even in disability rights movements, where in the past, insufficient attention has been paid to what access, inclusion, and equity might look like for those with more significant forms of intellectual disability (Finn et al. 2022, Jansen-van Vuuren and Aldersey 2020). This is beginning to evolve with the shift from disability rights to a disability justice framework: now, with the tenets of intersectionality being more seriously heeded, and where much work has been done to ensure that "no disability is left behind," folks are beginning to think more about equity for *all* forms of disability (McDonald et al. 2023, Peabody and Feinsinger 2024, Suarez-Balcazar et al. 2023). Still, there is still much work to be done, both practically and conceptually.

In the clinical care of non-speaking intellectually disabled patients, particularly those with more significant disabilities that preclude language-based forms of communication, clinicians are faced with uniquely challenging situations. Such patients not only lack the communicative capabilities to self-advocate, but it is also often unclear to what degree they comprehend the communicative acts of others or possess the capacity to participate in decisions regarding their care.

However, non-speaking intellectually disabled patients are not like others whose inability to participate fully in their healthcare emerges as a product of their individual bodymind. Children, for example, will become more immersed in language. Unlike those who have lost capacities that allow them to communicate effectively, such as patients with neurodegenerative diseases or those who have suffered brain injuries, they were never autonomous, independent communicators. And although the non-speaking intellectually disabled do comprise a vulnerable, oppressed group, the nature of their disabilities is distinct from other types of disabilities, in that ableism is not the primary barrier to equitable healthcare outcomes: the disability itself presents a distinct challenge to clinicians striving to meet the ideals of patient-centered communication because of the lack of access to linguistic forms of communication. Speaking to communicate never was, nor never will be possible, and amending forms of oppression will not alter the communicative challenges facing clinicians charged with their care. Typical medical training does not delve into the atypical means of communication more accessible to those with significant intellectual disabilities: the sorts of communication that might be employed by pairs of non-speaking intellectually disabled patients and their intimates are idiosyncratic and require individual attention to individual cases, rendering standardized training near impossible logistically.

Compounding the issue, the norms of patient-centered care for people with disabilities nonetheless require effective communication and compliance with the Americans with Disabilities Act. But how are clinicians with little experience with non-speaking intellectually disability to meet these requirements? The problems these clinician-patient pairs face have both a practical and systemic dimension.

At the practical level, imagine a typical encounter between a clinician and a patient. Clinicians typically work to discern a patient's agenda with open-ended questions. They (ideally) avoid jargon or interrupting the patient and they engage in focused, active listening.

In cases where communication or capacity is an issue, clinicians look to a caretaker, parent, or surrogate decision-maker. Lacking the presence of such a person, clinicians might try their best to quickly and effectively discern what a patient wants or needs. The standard constraints of HMO-based healthcare practices limit clinicians to 15-minute interactions per patient. However, without the expedience of linguistic communication, those with non-speaking intellectual disabilities likely require more substantive face-to-face time so that they can develop atypical modes of communication. But resource limitations often make it the case that clinicians are unable to devote additional time, and as such, healthcare outcomes can fall short of their potential.

The second, structural issue affects the nature of the care that intellectually disabled patients receive. Recent studies have shown that provider attitudes contribute to healthcare access and outcome disparity because of the way attitudes shape clinical decision-making (VanPuymbrouck et al. 2020, Iezzoni et al. 2021). These studies assessed disability in all its forms. Unfortunately, intellectual disability is sometimes the form of disability most affected by ableist attitudes, as is evidenced by continued problems with access in healthcare, education, living situation, job access, and so on. The conflation of the myriad forms of intellectual disability into the single cultural trope of the "r-word" has had horrific consequences for intellectually disabled people, who are often perceived as lacking a personality, individualized interests, or any complexity of inner life. What many people, including clinicians, lack is the sort of interpersonal relationships with a non-speaking intellectually disabled person that would allow them to see the fallaciousness of this belief.

One solution to the practical problem of communicating effectively, which could concurrently assuage concerns of implicit ableism, is the physical presence of a person who knows the intellectually disabled patient well during clinical encounters. The experiences of those close to these individuals suggest that plenty of non-language-based forms of communication do take place (Brison 2019; Crary 2018; Fleishmann & Fleishmann 2012; Goode 1994; Kittay 1999, 2009, 2019; Peabody Smith 2022). Further, the closer the relationship between those persons, the more successful interpretation will be. This has the potential to dramatically improve clinical outcomes because of the ability to more accurately discern the types of markers (like individual preference, autonomy, and personal values) that patient-centered care and communication endeavor to respect.

Of course, it is not always possible for an intimate of a non-speaking intellectually disabled person to be present during clinical encounters. Such a person does not always exist, and the presence of such a person, when they do exist, is not always permitted. When this is the case, we must rely on clinicians to do their utmost to communicate with this class of patients, despite their typical lack of training and experience.

David Goode's work in a rubella ward in the 1960s illustrates how this can occur in a clinical setting. Children affected by the Rubella epidemic of the 1960s were sometimes born deaf, blind, and intellectually disabled. Goode's work with these children highlights the ways in which unconventional forms of communication allowed such children to come to communicate with their caretakers (Goode 1994). When Goode began to focus his investigation on one child in the ward, a girl named Christina, he realized that working with individual children and fostering individual relationships would create an "opportunity to socially reconstruct [that child] in a fashion truer to their actual human qualities and capabilities" (Goode 1994, 17). Goode endeavored to establish the sort of close interpersonal relationship with Christina that would allow for the pair to understand one another in some meaningful sense.

Goode also studied another intellectually disabled and deaf-blind child, Bianca, who remained home with her family. In both cases, he observed unique communicative practices develop within the fiber of particular relationships. He noted that for Christina and Bianca, communication was available via touch, proprioception, and most significantly via "the engagement with their society that their senses and the structures of their societies permitted... through the mutual production and interpretation of 'indexical expressions'" (Goode 1994, 100), by which he means idiosyncratic communicative acts particular to small groups of users who rely on the context and history of a relationship to communicate.

Goode and Christina, as well as Bianca and her parents, were able to communicate with one another in various ways. For example, Goode would greet Christina by placing his hand on her face, and she would respond by gesturing to be picked up or by placing her right (less impaired) ear on his mouth, indicating she wanted him to sing to her (Goode 1994, 111). They were able to establish effective communication precisely because of the relationships that existed between the pairs. This corroborates the claim that the intimates of non-speaking intellectually disabled patients – pairs where relationships are preexisting – likely have privileged perspectives on the desires and needs of these individuals. They have already spent the necessary time together to develop the kinds of relationships required to communicate atypically and effectively.

To return to cases where practical constraints like time, the unavailability of such an intimate, or emergency conditions might affect care, consider what took place during the early phases of the COVID-19 pandemic. The nature of triage care had devastating effects on many disabled populations. Clinicians faced incredibly difficult decisions when allocating limited resources to overwhelming numbers of patients, each of whom presented life-threatening symptoms of a poorly understood virus. Further, in the early phases of COVID-19, some hospitals were limiting the permissibility of caregivers to be present with even non-speaking patients.

Denying non-speaking intellectually disabled patients an in-person advocate constitutes a particular form of healthcare injustice. It is a direct affront to the values of patient-centered communication, which for this group require either an in-person advocate or the time and resources necessary to develop effective communication. Because emergency conditions made it the case that the time was incredibly pressed for overwhelmed healthcare workers, the right to an in-person advocate for non-speaking patients must be protected in future emergency scenarios.

Much research has been conducted regarding triage care and disability, albeit in non-pandemic circumstances. As highlighted by a 2020 report by the National Council on Disability, the use of quality adjusted life years (QALYs) systematically devalues the lives of those with disabilities. QALYs are a commonly used economic metric in healthcare that are meant to compare the relative cost-effectiveness of different potential healthcare interventions. They are used by healthcare decision-makers and responsible parties (like insurance companies) to provide guidelines in triage settings and in non-emergency situations. To calculate the number of QALYs a certain intervention is expected to produce, one multiplies *expected years of life* by *health utility value*. Health utility value is a term used to capture a person's overall health-related quality of life, scaled from zero (dead) to one (perfect health). The way QALYs are calculated has a lot of problems (Cupples 2020; John, Millum, and Wasserman 2017; National Council on Disability 2022; Persad 2020; Whitehead and Ali 2010). The questionnaires used to determine health utility value are overly simplistic, failing to capture the way some symptoms may cross domains, the symptoms which matter more to certain patients, or the impact medications or assistive technologies might have on mitigating symptoms. There are issues with nuance: they can make disabilities look similar when they are not in fact similar. There are issues with application: the same survey results can be used for different purposes, and the same survey can have remarkably different outcomes. Finally, there are issues with imagination: it is difficult for a non-disabled person to imagine how their life would change with a disability, or what the lives of those with disabilities are in fact like.

This is why health utility values are a particular challenge when we turn to disability. One way of calculating health utility values involves asking members of the general population time trade-off questions, like "how many years of living with a particular disability would you trade for a shorter number of years spent in perfect health?" (National Council on Disability 2022). But these outcomes are based upon the perceptions of the non-disabled population. This means that non-disabled persons' biases and misperceptions of the quality of life of disabled people can have huge implications for the lives and treatment of disabled patients. Healthcare decision makers subsequently use the results of these types of surveys to assess the impact of disability on health, determining how much "worse" it is to be in a disabled condition than it is to be in a non-disabled one, as if this fundamentally subjective judgment could be evaluated objectively via empirical methods. Healthcare interventions for disabled patients typically have a lower comparable QALY-value and are thus deemed *not to be* as cost-effective.

During emergency conditions like the COVID-19 pandemic, this reasoning led to discrimination against disabled people and cost lives. Dr. Wendy Ross, director of the Center for Autism and Neurodiversity at Jefferson Health in Philadelphia, writes of the terrible toll the COVID-19 pandemic had on intellectually disabled patients, who were six times more likely than non-intellectually disabled patients to die from COVID-19. This was due at least in part to the fact that interventions for those with intellectual disabilities were deemed less cost-effective and to have a lower impact on improving quality of life than were interventions for non-disabled individuals (Ross 2021). Early in the pandemic, Alabama's guidelines – which were, fortunately, rescinded – allowed doctors to deny ventilator access to patients with intellectual disabilities, largely based upon the low numerical QALY outcome of ventilator use for this category of patient (Ross 2021). Dr. Ross suggests that although healthcare workers needed to limit visitors to reduce the spread of COVID-19, patients with intellectual disabilities need someone with them to communicate effectively or at all.

With the above in mind, I suggest two measures to protect patients with non-speaking intellectual disabilities. First, I argue that both the guidelines of patient-centered communication and the Americans with Disabilities Act (ADA) *require* that an in-person advocate be present, regardless of circumstances, for non-speaking intellectually disabled patients. Second, I will show how the application of a handicap system like the one used by golfers might improve QALY use overall in cases where disability is a factor.

The metrics that healthcare payers and providers rely upon consistently and systematically tell us that the lives of intellectually disabled patients are less worth saving than those of non-disabled ones. Because most clinicians lack the time, impetus, or resources necessary to work closely with non-speaking intellectually disabled patients in the way Goode was able to – particularly in triage settings – we must protect this already vulnerable patient population by insisting on their right to have an advocate present, or, when that is not an option, sufficient one-on-one time with a healthcare worker who can establish some form of communication. In future pandemic or pandemic-like circumstances, this right must be safeguarded. Like the ADA's protection of reasonable accommodations, the presence of an advocate (in the form of a family member, caretaker, friend, or even patient advocate) provides an accommodation for a non-speaking intellectually disabled individual in the medical setting. This does not present "undue hardship" so long as sensible protections, such as mask-wearing, social distancing, etc., are adhered to.

These are not the only ways to mitigate potential concerns of implicit ableism and their very real practical effects. If we have learned anything about this patient population from triage practices during the COVID-19 pandemic, it is that we must think ahead so that we can provide just healthcare, improved access, and fewer unwarranted deaths in future crises. Good solutions and decisions rarely emerge from conditions of duress, extreme stress, and a world in turmoil. So, given that many triage protocols were derived from a utilitarian, QALY-guided ethic, I want to suggest a way to improve the QALY calculus in order to get ahead of potential emergency conditions. (I make these suggestions with the caveat that, to my eye, QALYs are a far from ideal – and in fact, far from decent – metric. Nonetheless, insofar as they are the industry standard that responsible parties and healthcare economists rely upon to make difficult situations, I work to improve the actual as opposed to ideal world.)

So how might we improve QALY calculations in non-emergency conditions so that emergency protocols might derive from a place of justice-oriented considerations? Others have made suggestions, from using community-based participatory research as an empirical tool to inform health utility score calculations (Cupples 2020); to a "pathways approach" to setting triage priorities, where decision-makers could consider quality-of-life factors that are unavoidable results of a disability but *not* factors that are a result of discrimination or injustice (Persad 2019, 2020); to removing expected future *quality-of-life* considerations altogether from cost-effectiveness considerations, and instead focusing exclusively on life years gained (Persad, Wertheimer, and Emanuel 2010; Kerstein 2017). Many others either implicitly or explicitly endorse a view in which discrimination based on disability status can be justified in emergency conditions (Beckstead and Ord 2016; National Council on Disability 2020). Except for the final view, these are promising ideas, and I take myself to be adding to the potential solutions on the table as opposed to criticizing the measures suggested by the aforementioned.

With a nod to the irony of the nomenclature, I propose the application of a *handicap* to QALY calculations involving disabilities or other specific, small groups of the population. In the same way that golfers of varying levels apply a handicap to their final scores to attempt to level the playing field across different skill-levels and body types, decision-makers might integrate a similar strategy when evaluating the cost-effectiveness of various healthcare interventions or decision-making protocols in triage situations.

For example, imagine a case involving the expected cost-effectiveness of a liver transplant. A non-disabled person needing the transplant might have an expected outcome of 25 years of life gained with a health utility value of 0.75, so $25 \times 0.75 = 18.75$ QALYs would be gained were this patient granted the transplant. However, imagine another patient–one, for example, with autism. Healthcare decision-makers in this hypothetical case have conducted a time trade-off survey asking patients how many years with a moderate form of autism they would trade for non-autistic years, with the result being that, on average, those surveyed would trade 30 years with autism for 18 years without it. This yields a health utility value of 0.6. Assuming that the expected years of life gained with the liver transplant were the same, $25 \times 0.6 = 15$

QALYs would be gained by the autistic potential recipient. The non-disabled patient would receive the liver.

Now, were decision-makers to integrate a handicap system like the one used by golfers, the playing field might become a bit more leveled. Say they were required to apply some kind of system to QALY calculations involving health utility scores derived from time trade-off surveys when those surveys involved disabilities. Responsible parties, stakeholders, and health-care decision-makers could deliberate to agree upon exact numbers, but we could imagine them deciding that health utility scores involving moderate intellectual disabilities would receive a 0.15 handicap. This would, of course, by contingent upon the identification of sub-classes of intellectual disability (for example, as is being attempted in current precision health-care research involving the identification of subclasses of autism). Distinct subclasses or diagnoses could receive different handicaps, determined by principles of equal access, justice, proportional social disadvantage, etc. Applying this to the above case, the health utility value for the patient with autism would increase to 0.75, and were they to receive the liver transplant, the number of QALYs gained would be **25 × 0.75 = 18.75**: the same as the non-disabled one. Given that, on average, disabled individuals rate their quality of life similarly to non-disabled individuals and given that many disabilities do not bear direct implications on other aspects of health or upon overall health, *this outcome makes more sense than the assumptions made by non-disabled time trade-off survey takers.*

Further, we can imagine how time trade-off surveys might particularly denigrate non-speaking intellectually disabled conditions. Many of us would sacrifice many years to avoid such a state. Our assessments of time-tradeoffs for conditions of mind so wholly unimaginable to the non-intellectually disabled would likely be influenced by implicitly ableist beliefs, failures of imagination, fear, and the like: these are all, of course, appropriate reactions to this bizarre form of imaginative reasoning, which is further reason to avoid the use of time trade-off questioning in the development and deployment of cost-effectiveness models. So, agreeing on a handicap point system that more aptly captures the fact that quality of life is not neces-sarily low for such persons might protect their lives and access to healthcare. While my exam-ple QALY calculations have been simplistic, we can see how the application of a handicap might aid in assuaging the ableist underpinnings of QALY use in both emergency and non-emergency contexts. Especially for patients incapable of self-advocacy, the institution of a more just calculus that protects access to limited resources is pressing. This would allow healthcare workers and other stakeholders to more earnestly apply the principles of patient-centered communication to a class of patients where communicating is particularly challeng-ing and in cases where resources are intensely strained. The type of outcome disparities witnessed in COVID-19 cannot occur again, insofar as we are committed to healthcare justice for all patients.

Work Cited

Beckstead, Nick and Toby Ord. 2016. "Bubbles under the Wallpaper: Healthcare Rationing and Discrimination." In *Bioethics: An Anthology*, 3rd ed, edited by Helga Kuhse, Udo Schüklenk & Peter Singer, 406–412. Hoboken, NJ: Wiley.

Brison, Susan. 2019. "Foreword" In *Learning from My Daughter: The Value and Care of Disabled Minds*, Eva Feder Kittay, xi–xvii. Oxford: Oxford University Press.

Campbell, Stephen M. & Stramondo, Joseph A. 2017. "The Complicated Relationship of Disability and Well-Being." *Kennedy Institute of Ethics Journal* 27 (2): 151–184.

Crary, Alice. 2018. "The Horrific History of Comparisons between Cognitive Disability and Animality (and How to Move Past It)." In *Animalidies: Gender, Animals, and Madness*, edited by Lori Gruen and Fiona Probyn-Rapsey, 117–136. New York: Bloomsbury.

Cupples, Laura. 2020. "Disability, Epistemic Harms, and the Quality-Adjusted Life Year." *International Journal of Feminist Approaches to Bioethics* 13: 45–62.

Diab Marguerite E., and Mark V. Johnston. 2004. "Relationships between Level of Disability and Receipt of Preventive Health Services." *Archives of Physical Medicine and Rehabilitation* 85 (5): 749–57. https://doi.org/10.1016/j.apmr.2003.06.028

Epstein, Ronald M., and Richard L. Street, Jr. 2011. "The Values and Value of Patient-centered Care." *Annals of Family Medicine* 9 (2): 100–103.

Ervin, David A., Brian Hennen, Joav Merrick, and Mohammed Morad. 2014. "Healthcare for Persons with Intellectual and Developmental Disability in the Community." *Frontiers in Public Health* 2: 83.

Finn, Chester A., Matthew S. Smith, Michael Ashley Stein. 2022. "How Persons with Intellectual Disabilities Are Fighting for Decision-Making Rights." *Current History* 121 (831): 30–35.

Fix, Gemmae M., Carol VanDeusen Lukas, Rendelle E. Bolton, Jennifer N. Hill, Nora Mueller, Sherri L. LaVela, and Barbara G. Bokhour. 2018. "Patient-centred Care is a Way of Doing Things: How Healthcare Employees Conceptualize Patient-centred Care." *Health Expectations* 21 (1): 300–307.

Fleishmann, Arthur and Carly Fleishmann. 2012. *Carly's Voice: Breaking Through Autism*. New York: Touchstone.

Goode, David. 1994. *A World Without Words: The Social Construction of Children Born Deaf and Blind*. Philadelphia: Temple University Press.

Kerstein, Samuel. 2017. "Dignity, Disability, and Lifespan." *Journal of Applied Philosophy* 34 (5): 635–650. https://doi.org/10.1111/japp.12158

Kittay, Eva Feder. 1999. *Love's Labor*. New York: Routledge.

Kittay, Eva Feder. 2019. *Learning from My Daughter*. Oxford: Oxford University Press.

Kittay, Eva Feder. 2009. "The Personal is Philosophical is Political: A Philosopher and Mother of a Cognitively Disabled Person Sends Notes from the Battlefield." *Metaphilosophy* 40: 606–627.

Krahn, Gloria L., Deborah Klein Walker, and Rosaly Correa-De-Araujo. 2015. "Persons with disabilities as an unrecognized health disparity population." *American Journal of Public Health* 105 (Suppl 2): S198–S206. https://doi.org/10.2105/AJPH.2014.302182

Iezzoni, Lisa I., Sowmya R Rao, Julie Ressalam, Dragana Bolcic-Jankovic, Nicole D Agaronnik, Karen Donelan, Tara Lagu, and Eric G Campbell. 2021. "Physicians' Perceptions of People with Disability and Their Health Care." *Health Affairs* 40 (2): 297–306.

Inclusion International. 2020. *Excluded from the Excluded: People with Intellectual Disabilities in (and out of) Official Development Assistance*. London: Inclusion International. https://inclusion-international. org/resource/excluded-from-the-excluded-people-with-intellectual-disabilities-in-and-out-of-official-development-assistance/

Jansen-van Vuuren, J., & Aldersey, H. M. 2020. "Stigma, Acceptance and Belonging for People with IDD Across Cultures." *Current Developmental Disorders Reports* 7 (3): 163–172. https://doi. org/10.1007/s40474-020-00206-w

John, T.M., Millum, J., and Wasserman, D. 2017. "How to Allocate Scarce Health Resources Without Discriminating Against People with Disabilities." *Economics and Philosophy* 33 (2): 161–184.

Persad, Govind, Alan Wertheimer and Ezekiel J. Emanuel. 2010. "Standing by Our Principles: Meaningful Guidance, Moral Foundations, and Multi-Principle Methodology in Medical Scarcity." *American Journal of Bioethics* 10 (4): 46–48.

McDonald, Katherine E., Ariel E. Schwartz, Micah Fialka Feldman, Tia Nelis, and Dora M. Raymaker. 2023. "A Call-In for Allyship and Anti-Ableism in Intellectual Disability Research." *American Journal on Intellectual and Developmental Disability* 128 (6): 398–410. https://doi.org/10.1352/1944-7558-128.6.398

National Council on Disability. "Policy Brief: Alternatives to QALY-based Cost-Effectiveness for Determining the Value of Prescription Drugs and Other Health Interventions." November 28, 2022. Accessed 8/6/24. https://www.ncd.gov/assets/uploads/reports/2022/ncd_alternatives_to_the_qaly_508.pdf

Okoro, Catherine A., NaTasha D. Hollis, Alissa C. Cyrus, and Shannon Griffin-Blake. 2018. "Prevalence of Disabilities and Health Care Access by Disability Status and Type among Adults—United States, 2016." *Morbidity and Mortality Weekly Reports* 67 (32): 882–887. https://doi.org/10.15585/mmwr. mm6732a3

Peabody Smith, Ally. 2022. "How Should (and Shouldn't) We Think about Profound Intellectual Disability?" *Journal of Philosophy of Disability* 2: 112–129.

Peabody Smith A. and Ashley Feinsinger. 2024. "Extending Patient-centred Communication to Non-speaking Intellectually Disabled Persons." *Journal of Medical Ethics* Online First. https://doi.org/10.1136/jme-2023-109671

Persad, G. 2019. "Considering Quality of Life while Repudiating Disability Injustice: A Pathways Approach to Setting Priorities." *The Journal of Law, Medicine & Ethics* 47 (2): 294–303.

Persad, G. 2020. "The Pathways Approach to Priority Setting: Considering Quality of Life While Being Fair to Individuals with Disabilities." In *Disability, Health, Law, and Bioethics*, edited by I. Cohen, C. Shachar, A. Silvers, & M. Stein, 255–265. Cambridge: Cambridge University Press.

Reynolds, April. 2009. "Patient-centered Care." *Radiologic Technology* 81 (2): 133–147.

Ross, Wendy. 2021. "The terrible toll of COVID-19 on people with intellectual disabilities." *Association of American Medical Colleges*, April 20, 2021. https://www.aamc.org/news-insights/terrible-toll-covid-19-people-intellectual-disabilities

Santana, Maria J., Kimberly Manalili, Rachel J Jolley, Sandra Zelinsky, Hude Quan, Mingshan Lu. 2018. "How to Practice Person-Centred Care: A Conceptual Framework." *Health Expectations* 21 (2): 429–440.

Suarez-Balcazar, Yolanda, Fabricio Balcazar, Delphine Labbe, Katherine E. McDonald, Christopher Keys, Tina Taylor-Ritzler, Sarah M. Anderson, and Joy Agner. 2023. "Disability Rights and Empowerment: Reflections on AJCP Research and a Call to Action." *American Journal of Community Psychology* 72: 317–327.

VanPuymbrouck, Laura, Carli Friedman, and Heather Feldner. 2020. "Explicit and Implicit Disability Attitudes of Healthcare Providers." *Rehabilitation Psychology* 65 (2): 101–112.

Whitehead, S.J., and Ali, S. 2010. "Health Outcomes in Economic Evaluation: The QALY and Utilities." *British Medical Bulletin* 96: 5–21. https://doi.org/10.1093/bmb/ldq033

World Health Organization. 2016. *Patient engagement. technical series on safer primary care*. Geneva: World Health Organization.

PART III

Before the Next Pandemic

8

LONG COVID AND DISABILITY JUSTICE

Critiquing the Present, Forming the Future

Sarah Clark Miller

Temporalities of Pandemic Harm: Complicating Before and After Narratives

In distinguishing the concepts of debilitation and disablement in *The Right to Maim*, Jasbir Puar (2017) writes:

> I contend that the term 'debilitation' is distinct from the term 'disablement' because it fore-grounds the slow wearing down of populations instead of the event of becoming disabled. While the latter concept creates and hinges on a narrative of before and after for individuals who will eventually be identified as disabled, the former comprehends those bodies that are sustained in a perpetual state of debilitation precisely through foreclosing the social, cultural, and political translation to disability.
>
> *(xiii–xiv)*

The narrative structure of an event—of a before and an after—that Puar identifies as characteristic of disablement strongly informs cultural conversations surrounding COVID, yet in ways that offer simultaneous resonance with and distinction from Puar's framework. Consideration of the growing global prevalence of long COVID in conversation with the conceptual resources found in Puar's discussions of debilitation and disablement prove indispensable for better grasping and responding to ongoing pandemic harms.

The cultural framing of SARS-CoV-2 infection largely follows a before-and-after narrative not of disablement but of cure: people get COVID, are sick for a discrete period of time, and then recover (Clare 2017). The "after" of COVID is predominantly understood to be one of returning to the baseline condition of how one was prior to infection. The emergence of the post-viral syndrome of long COVID[1] complicated the narrative structure of cure. We began to realize that after a SARS-CoV-2 infection, some experienced long COVID (even sometimes after believing themselves to have been mostly cured). Long COVID thus represents an alternative kind of after—not of cure, but rather a medical, social, and political state of limbo.

In the *alternative after* of long COVID, as we might call it, the foreclosing of the social, cultural, and political translation to disability characteristic of debility appears, but for

DOI: 10.4324/9781003502623-12

reasons and in ways not fully emblematic of Puar's concept of debility. Puar (2017) reserves the term "debility" to "[address] injury and bodily exclusion that are endemic rather than epidemic or exceptional," and clearly, the origins of long COVID are epidemic (xvii). In that the origins are epidemic, on Puar's account, long COVID should be considered to be a form of disability. Moreover, the slow wearing down of populations emblematic of debility does not resonate with how long COVID arises. Yet, Puar also advances the concept of debility "to illuminate the possibilities and limits of disability imaginaries and economies" (xvi). The emergence of accurate medical and political understandings of long COVID has required an expansion of disability imaginaries and economies, as the intense struggles for "a legitimate identification with disability that is manifest through state, market, and institutional recognition" illustrate (xiv). In order to conceptualize long COVID as a form of disability, societies first must be willing to acknowledge—politically and medically—that long COVID is real, is widespread, and is here to stay. Such beliefs have been tough to secure.

COVID narratives also display how the temporality of pandemic harms tends to split into two distinct durations: the swift strike of being felled by SARS-CoV-2 contrasted with the gaping expanse of long COVID. Before, one version of the story goes, people were healthy. After being infected with SARS-CoV-2 and after the acute phase of COVID-19, while most recover, some remained sick, indefinitely impaired—systems not functioning the way they used to. In the temporally expansive *alternative after* of long COVID, where clear thinking once reigned, there is brain fog. Where the steady rhythm of a heart was, tuplets or too much speed appear. Where once there were reliable vein thoroughfares, now there are dangerous clots and blockages.

Narratives can be elegant in their explanatory power. But from the start, we need to treat them with some suspicion—intentionally complicating aspects that seem too pat. While in certain cases such narratives are accurate, they can also occlude other realities: many people live with forms of chronic illness and disability that heighten the dangers of the initial impact of the virus, the chances that they make it through alive, and the probability that an initial infection will result in long-haul symptoms. The point here is not to draw a bright line between chronically ill and disabled folks who cannot afford to get COVID and the rest of a robust, healthy population that can. Long COVID can take hold in those not previously disabled or ill, just as it can in those with preexisting conditions. The point, instead, is to make visible extant forms of chronic illness and disability that preceded the pandemic and that interact with COVID-19 in perilous ways.

Another series of factors that trouble before-and-after narratives arise in those who believed themselves to have recovered completely from COVID only to later find themselves with new maladies. Recently, for example, awareness of cases of cancer following SARS-CoV-2 infection has increased. In May 2023, health writer Lisa Mulcahy (2023) reported that

[a] study from researchers at Mount Sinai Hospital in New York City, along with Universidade Estadual do Maranhão, Centro Universitário Christus, and Universidade Federal do Ceará in Brazil, described how, after recovering from COVID, previously healthy young adults were diagnosed, respectively, with acute myeloid leukemia, T-cell lymphoblastic leukemia and myelodysplastic syndrome, which turns into acute myeloid leukemia about 50% of the time.[2]

In this kind of case, yet another curious pandemic temporality of harm evidences itself: one in which there are those who believed themselves to have entered an "after" of cure and health rather than disablement, only later to discover that COVID dealt them delayed, long-term harm.

Long COVID as a Mass Disabling Event

Alongside the before-and-after narratives of COVID we now find a second story that few want to hear: the COVID-19 pandemic is a mass disabling event. While many wish to ignore such a claim and the emerging reality it ushers in as they rush to return to "normal," the numbers support the credibility of this claim. The American Academy of Physical Medicine and Rehabilitation (AAPM&R) estimates that as of the end of January 2023, 30,166,231 of the 100,554,103 cases of COVID Americans have experienced have resulted in Post-Acute Sequelae of SARS-CoV-2 infection (PASC) or long COVID ("PASC Dashboard"). This calculation assumes that 30% of those Americans who survive COVID-19 end up with long COVID. As journalist Benjamin Mazer (2022), writing for the *Atlantic*, points out, the assumptions that produce this calculation "may be a major undercount" because the count represents confirmed cases of COVID in the United States. The Household Pulse Survey, run by the National Center for Health Statistics in partnership with the Census Bureau, estimated that as of January 2023, 15.1% of all adults in the United States had experienced long COVID—nearly one in six adults (National Center for Health Statistics). The percentage of adults in the United States with long COVID is thought to have reduced and stabilized in 2024, as

> 7% of all adults…reported currently having long COVID in March 2024. The latest data show that rates of long COVID have remained relatively consistent for the last year, suggesting they may persist indefinitely unless new forms of prevention or treatment are discovered.
>
> *(Burns 2024)*

The percentage of people who develop long COVID may ultimately be higher—20%? (Ducharme 2022; Lara Bull-Otterson, et al. 2022) 30%? (WebMD Editorial Contributors 2022) More than 50%? (Cox 2021; Groff et al. 2021).

While the sheer magnitude of such numbers is regrettably striking, their noteworthiness needs to be considered in an extended historical trajectory. Members of the Long COVID Justice Project remind us that "[l]ong COVID is just the most recent manifestation of a long under-acknowledged phenomenon of post-infection illness that often drives, worsens, or unmasks a set of understudied complex chronic conditions" (Long COVID Justice Project). Moreover, COVID is far from the first pandemic in recent years to reveal "the critical need for large-scale change in healthcare, public health, and unjust structures that bring inequitable risks of illness, suffering, and mortality" (Long COVID Justice Project). The HIV/AIDS pandemic exposed related fracture lines in healthcare systems, as well as the presence of violence and systemic oppression for vulnerable populations.

As long COVID continues to confound medical practitioners, some are realizing they can borrow aspects of the treatment playbook from related post-viral illnesses such as myalgic encephalomyelitis and post-treatment Lyme disease syndrome (Choutka et al. 2022). It is also important to note that long COVID has sometimes shared with those diseases being on the receiving end of medicine's skepticism (Lowe 2022). Forms of disbelief that reduce long COVID to a series of psychosomatic symptoms exacerbate the problem of achieving societal recognition of the extensive (not to mention real) nature of the problem. In addition, the connection between long COVID and other viral-onset conditions needs to be amplified, not only to possibly generate swifter and more perceptive medical research but also for reasons of fostering better knowledge transfer from those who have been living with chronic illness for years to those who have newly joined the ranks.

Four-plus years since the beginning of COVID pandemic, an unfulfilled and crucial moral and political imperative persists: to acknowledge that the original waves of the COVID-19 emergency have given rise to the very real worldwide disablement of a substantial number of those who initially contracted SARS-CoV-2 and now need various forms of medical, economic, and social support. Long COVID is nothing less than a slow-burning global health crisis with implications that arc far into the future (Faghy et al. 2022). Acknowledgment of and response to long COVID is a moral imperative because the harms to those with long COVID, to their families, and to the many relationships with friends, colleagues, and communities that falter in the face of chronic illness continue to mount. Acknowledgment of and response to long COVID is a political imperative because it will take collective political will (or at least broad swaths of support) to establish the response long COVID sufferers need and to slow down the runaway train that began when many governments dropped COVID mitigation practices.

While scientific research and opinion regarding the scope of long COVID has shifted somewhat as the pandemic has continued to evolve, the scope of disablement remains astonishing. A March 2023 editorial in *The Lancet* observes:

> Although the majority of patients infected with SARS-CoV-2 recover within a few weeks, long COVID is estimated to occur in 10-20% of cases and affects people of all ages, including children, with most cases occurring in patients with mild acute illness. The consequence is widespread global harm to people's health, wellbeing, and livelihoods…
>
> *(Lancet 2023, 795)*[3]

Recent estimates put the global toll of long COVID at upwards of 65 million people—"based on a conservative estimated incidence of 10% of infected people and more than 651 million documented COVID-19 cases worldwide" (Davis et al. 2023, 134). That's at least 65 million people who experience a selection from a growing catalog of over 200 possible symptoms for at least months and sometimes years. Tens of millions of people worldwide have had their health and well-being permanently altered by long COVID.

To detractors who would object that the heightened concern regarding the global impact of long COVID on health and wellbeing is overblown, one might say the following: At the very least, long COVID represents an ongoing mass disabling event of a temporary nature. At a minimum, long COVID limits the daily activities of those who suffer from it for a period of months. This in and of itself should be cause for concern. Yet, while there is evidence that some recover from long COVID, for others, symptoms undoubtedly persist. Moreover, as the pandemic rattles on, the risks of experiencing long COVID mount. SARS-CoV-2 variants continue to evolve and tumble onto the scene, infecting and reinfecting people. With each successive infection, the risk of experiencing long COVID increases (Schmidt 2023). Moreover, those whose immune response has been compromised by long COVID are more likely to get infected again. All of this is to say that absent better forms of treatment, we can, unfortunately, predict the continued disabling of the world's population via long COVID.

Before turning to the essential question of how to map a better response to long COVID, there is one final point regarding the health and diagnostic disparities that are the predictable results of systemic racism and economic disadvantage. We have known for a while that disparities exist in how people of color have, on the whole, fared worse than their white counterparts during the pandemic in terms of experiencing higher rates of COVID-19, higher rates of hospitalization, and higher mortality rates as a result of COVID-19 (Ndugga, Hill, and Artiga 2022). Certain impacts of oppression increase risks of mortality in the acute phases of COVID-19. Predictably, recent studies have shown that health disparities pertain not only to COVID but also to long COVID. A study published in February 2023 demonstrated that in days 31–180 following infection, Black patients (both hospitalized and non-hospitalized) developed new illnesses, including diabetes, pulmonary embolism, and headaches more often than white patients. Hispanic patients (both hospitalized and non-hospitalized) developed chest pain, headaches, and dyspnea more frequently than white patients (Khullar et al. 2023).

Furthermore, other studies demonstrate that "the population of patients diagnosed with ['Post COVID-19 condition, unspecified'] is demographically skewed toward female, White, non-Hispanic individuals, as well as individuals living in areas with low poverty and low unemployment" (Pfaff et al. 2023). There is little surprise that those with greater resources and easier access to healthcare are those who are able to receive long COVID diagnoses, thereby unlocking at least some care for their ongoing condition. Once long COVID is on the scene, some populations will receive frequent and thorough medical attention, while other populations are more likely to languish—cut off from the care needed to facilitate recovery. Any discussions of experiences pre- and post-COVID must take into account various vectors of privilege that shape the episodes of both acute and chronic illness.

Long COVID and Disability Justice in and Beyond Emergency Conditions

While many people, institutional entities, and governments have declared the pandemic over, long COVID represents the reality of the mass disabling power of SARS-CoV-2. The magnitude of this situation, when mixed with divisive politics and institutions already infused with ableism, racism, classism, and sexism, has resulted in outright denial and wildly inadequate care, that is, when care can be found at all. This is to say that just as the harms of the early emergency conditions of the early pandemic years were best understood through an intersectional lens, the mass disabling event that long COVID is, now that the emergency conditions of COVID have purportedly receded, must also be understood as a complex set of interlocking injustices.

A series of pivotal questions arises in the face of these interlocking injustices: What exactly has gone wrong thus far? How do we best articulate and explain the key failures? How might we more clearly perceive the moral, social, and political harms of long COVID? In addition, we also need to ask: What would a better response—an adequate one, let alone an ideal one—to long COVID look like? How can we envision a future that affords all long haulers not only adequate medical treatment but also robust social support and care?

One of the richest sources of expertise when wishing to analyze the major missteps vis-à-vis long COVID, as well as to bring forth a vision of alternative futures, is the community of disability justice activists and scholars. What can disability justice scholars teach us about how to shift societal understandings of and responses to long COVID? In what follows, I turn to Leah Lakshmi Piepzna-Samarasinha and Mia Mingus for tools to critique of the myriad failures of current responses to long COVID. Critical examination of the present can clear a path for envisioning better futures. Amplification and expansion of the "Ten Principles of Disability Justice" from Sins Invalid helps lead the way.

Critiquing Present Failures

In *Care Work*, Leah Lakshmi Piepzna-Samarasinha (2018) identifies a model of care they call "the crash and burn emergency model" (52). Emergency-response care webs—the kinds of webs that the crash and burn emergency model generates—arise when an able-bodied person becomes disabled (temporarily or permanently), usually through injury or acute illness. A rapid mobilization of their able-bodied community occurs in response to the crisis. As Piepzna-Samarasinha characterizes it: "There are emails and calls and care calendars set up, and (mostly able-bodied) people show up to the hospital. (Mostly able-bodied) people cook food and throw benefits. There's a sense of urgency! Purpose! Action! OMG, someone is sick! We must come together as a community to help them!" (52) Piepzna-Samarasinha makes two sharp observations about such emergency-response care webs. First, when it is their (as Piepzna-Samarasinha puts it) "mountain-climbing friend who gets hit riding their bike," the able-body community cares deeply (52). But when it is people who have long lived with disabilities, care from such able-bodied communities is largely absent. Second, if the person who was injured or ill does not recover, hence coming to experience a long-term disability, the emergency-response care web unravels. What initially seemed like an urgent, individual problem is revealed instead to be one situated squarely amid the structural injustice of ableism and the institutional barriers it erects. Absent the buffer that emergency-response care webs can provide against experiences of ableism, those with long-term disabilities come face-to-face with the harsh realities of ongoing existence in a world designed to leave them behind.

Piepzna-Samarasinha's observations in 2018 proved prescient for the pandemic and long COVID. When the first wave of the virus hit, there was significant community urgency around responding to the many people who got sick. Friends and neighbors built care networks to deliver groceries and medicines to the doorsteps of those too sick and contagious to go out. These emergency-response care networks also began to meet the needs of people not currently sick with COVID but experiencing other pandemic-induced needs. Neighbors shared tips regarding where to find difficult-to-locate comestibles (broccoli was a favorite in my community) and other suddenly absent essentials (toilet paper seemed to be universally scarce). Clearly, the care webs that the emergency model generated weren't without value. But they also weren't well-sustained. There was community and coming together when COVID was novel, and its long-term implications were not well understood. As the pandemic wore on, those emergency-response care webs wore thin.

Piepzna-Samarasinha's criticism finds its greatest purchase in foretelling the way emergency-response care networks have faded in the presence of long COVID. Many in the group for whom COVID-19 was slow to recede have witnessed the crash and burn of the emergency COVID care their communities initially offered. As their illness continued, often morphing into new forms of malady and dysfunction, they found themselves increasingly isolated and ignored. They received less care right as they were being subjected to the ableism of the everyday world.

When those who were principally able-bodied before the pandemic suffer from long COVID, they come to experience first-hand the forms of structural injustice and institutional barriers ableism inflicts that have long been the persistent backdrop of disabled communities. These experiences, Mia Mingus (2022) argues, are shot through with abled supremacy, abled privilege, and ableist ignorance:

> Abled supremacy means that many of you mistakenly think that if you do get COVID and if you end up with long COVID, that the state will take care of you or that your community will. You believe this because you do not know about the lived reality of disability in this country. Abled privilege means that you don't have to listen to disabled people or learn about ableism and abled supremacy. Our government does not care about the disabled people that already exist. So, if you think it will care for you if you become disabled from COVID, as millions more will, then that is a function of your ableist ignorance.

People with disabilities knew that governmental institutions would be unlikely to provide adequate support for long COVID. Abled supremacy has never been a luxury they could afford. The millions of people with long COVID are perhaps beginning to understand the importance of moving beyond abled privilege in the specific form of learning from disabled people who have experienced ableism throughout their lives. Ultimately, for Mingus, the initial belief that the state would care for long haulers was emblematic of wider patterns of ableist ignorance.

While Mingus and Piepzna-Samarasinha advance different criticisms, they reach a similar conclusion in light of their critiques: those whose lives were previously not ruled by ableism—those who lived lives of abled-bodied privilege prior to long COVID—ought to listen to and learn from people with disabilities. Within Mingus's critique is an implicit call to dismantle abled supremacy and the abled privilege and ignorance that sustains it. Piepzna-Samarasinha, for their part, concludes that the crash and burn emergency model of care has "a lot to learn from disability justice models of centering sustainability, slowness, and building for the long haul" (Piepzna-Samarasinha 2018, 53). Holding Mingus and Piepzna-Samarasinha's critical engagements with the present and recent past in mind, I turn next to the "Ten Principles of Disability Justice" from Sins Invalid (2018) for insight regarding how to map a more promising future for long haulers.

Envisioning Possible Futures

In the "Ten Principles of Disability Justice," Patricia Berne (2018), on behalf of Sins Invalid, characterizes disability justice as "a vision and practice of a *yet-to-be...*" (229). The critical insights of disability justice scholars such as Mingus and Piepzna-Samarasinha make it clear that the present circumstances of long COVID are not sustainable. The Ten Principles lead us in the direction of what a better future for people with long COVID can be in the space of what is yet to be. While all ten principles offer potential insights for understanding and responding to long COVID, four of them seem particularly perspicacious as the mass disabling event of long COVID continues to unfold.[4] These four principles are Collective Liberation, Commitment to Cross-Disability Solidarity, Cross-Movement Organizing, and Leadership of Those Most Impacted.

The expanded description of the tenth principle, Collective Liberation, states, "[w]e move together as people with mixed abilities, multiracial, multi-gendered, mixed class, across the sexual spectrum, with a vision that leaves no bodymind behind" (229). Liberation within a disability justice framework requires the collective movement forward of people with varying and intersecting identities. From this, we glean that any possible vision of a better future for those with long COVID must cut across lines of able-bodiedness, race, class, gender, and sexuality. Any plan that moves the already privileged and relatively powerful ahead at the expense of others who are more socially vulnerable will be unacceptable. Moreover, the principle of Collective Liberation points out that such an approach simply won't be successful.

The building of solidarity must also happen within and across communities of people with disabilities. The seventh principle, Commitment to Cross-Disability Solidarity, calls for "building a movement that breaks down isolation," thus establishing greater connection between various experiences of disability, including physical disabilities, psychiatric disability, neurodiversity, and chronic illness (228). For Sins Invalid (2015), Commitment to Cross-Disability Solidarity is ultimately a commitment to valuing and honoring "the insights and participation of all of our community members, even and especially those who are most often left out of political conversations." Intentional building of cross-disability solidarity will involve the recognition that those who were disabled before the pandemic have similar concerns to those newly disabled with long COVID. It will also involve the recognition that those who were disabled before experiencing long COVID are sometimes most seriously affected by the condition. The societal response to long COVID needs to prioritize support not only for those newly disabled with long COVID but for all people with disabilities, and needs, in general, to conceptualize long COVID in relation to other forms of disability. The fight for a better future for those with long COVID ultimately must be a fight for a better future for all people with disabilities.

The fourth principle, Cross-Movement Solidarity (or Commitment to Cross-Movement Organizing),[5] reminds us of how essential it is to foster connection and solidarity between long haulers and those involved in other justice and liberation movements. Any single experience of long COVID will, of course, be situated within a network of relative privilege and oppression determined by several vectors (represented in another of the Ten Principles, Intersectionality). The Long COVID Justice Project demonstrates the importance of this principle in noting that "[d]isproportionate rates and impacts of disability and chronic illness are driven by the ongoing structural marginalization of Black, Brown and indigenous people, immigrants, queer and trans people, older people, poor and low-income people, those who are imprisoned and those without access to stable housing" (Long COVID Justice Project). While weathering long COVID is always difficult, that difficulty increases significantly when multiple forms of oppression interact, heightening disadvantage in general and the effects of illness and disability, more specifically.

Cross-movement organizing is all the more necessary given the shockingly insufficient state-level response to COVID and, now, to long COVID. Cross-movement organizing means organizing care in the face of state neglect, and, even worse, in the face of the wrongful, intentional harm governments exhibit when they believe those with chronic illnesses and disabilities hinder capitalism's imperative of economic progress. In "You Are Not Entitled to Our Deaths: COVID, Abled Supremacy & Interdependence," which Mia Mingus wrote in early 2022 after watching the state steamroll over human needs and lives for two long pandemic years, she remonstrates: "We will not look away from the mass illness and death that surrounds us or from a state machine that is more committed to churning out profit and privileged comfort with eugenic abandonment." Governments sacrificed the lives of high-risk individuals on the altar of late capitalism by failing to foster adequate protection for vulnerable populations (e.g., the elderly and those with preexisting conditions known to interact poorly with SARS-CoV-2) during the initial waves of COVID, as Mingus argues.

With long COVID, the logic is perhaps slightly different since "the vulnerable" do not comprise a discrete population to be sacrificed. When it comes to long COVID, we're all vulnerable. An abiding commitment to build cross-movement solidarity represents a necessary response to state acts of omission and commission, in order to ensure not only that long haulers receive adequate care but also that the availability of that care does not fall along all-too-predictable lines of race and class privilege. Beyond the neglect of state systems ill-equipped to respond well to a pandemic and state prioritization of profit over vulnerable lives, lies a suspicion even more grim and bleak. Mingus (2022) writes, "[w]e know we need systemic change so that our peoples can *literally* survive this pandemic, but we also know that the kind of changes we need are most likely not coming. It is in the interest of those in power to keep people uncared for, sick and dependent on dwindling crumbs." What circumstances would ensure the steady production of the inadequately cared for chronically ill, who are necessarily dependent on scanty state resources to survive? Long COVID certainly would. Solidarity between those working for justice on different fronts is perhaps the only way to respond to the intentional creation and maintenance of such precarity. (Mingus reminds us that both state-level and community support are ultimately needed; the latter is just more likely to emerge.) When the changes necessary for populations to better survive long COVID may not be coming from the level of the state, mechanisms of care can be built collectively between movements. At the same time, the political and economic forces keen to produce and maintain sickly and dependent populations reach well beyond the issue of long COVID. Multiple justice movements seek to liberate populations predictably rendered vulnerable and needy, be it for economic, health, or identity-based reasons. Solidarity around these linked forms of oppression can combat injustice more effectively.

Finally, the principle of Leadership of Those Most Impacted reminds us that we should prioritize the knowledge of long haulers by "lifting up, listening to, reading, following, and highlighting the perspective of those who are most impacted" both by long COVID and by the systems that have made recognition and treatment of this condition very difficult (Sins Invalid 2015). When faced with the denial that long COVID was a legitimate medical condition, long haulers stepped over the barriers medical experts' disbelief produced by organizing to generate and disseminate knowledge among long haulers themselves. In doing so, they lent one another epistemic weight. The concept of leadership in play in this principle is broadly construed and embraces cross-disability solidarity by welcoming the relevant expertise arising from related communities, as well. The Long COVID Justice Project serves as an excellent example of this kind of work in seeking to "center, platform, and resource those with Long COVID, complex chronic illnesses, and other disabilities at the forefront of policy, advocacy, and action related to these issues." A concrete example of such work is the petition the Long COVID Justice Project organized that urged the National Institutes of Health not to conduct planned long COVID clinical trials focused on exercise therapy. Long haulers and patient advocates emphasized that about half of all people with long COVID also have myalgic encephalomyelitis/chronic fatigue syndrome, making exercise-focused therapies potentially harmful for them. Initiatives like this petition highlight the importance of embracing the principle of Leadership of Those Most Impacted.

In *The Future Is Disabled*, Piepzna-Samarasinha (2022) introduces the concept of "crip doulaing," which directly amplifies the principle of Leadership of Those Most Impacted by emphasizing the vital knowledge transfer between those who have been around the block and the newly initiated. In discussing how the future is disabled, they write:

> There will be (already is) a need for crip doulaing on a massive scale, linking newly disabled people living with long COVID with people who have been sick and disabled longer, sharing our skills in living with chronic illness and fighting the medical industrial complex. In particular there are people in [the] chronic illness community, like folks living with CFIDS and MCS and late-stage Lyme, who have done community research on post-viral syndrome that millions of people living with long COVID desperately need. Our disabled histories of activism and survival skills are crucially needed—and most people outside disabled / chronically ill community don't know they exist.
>
> *(327)*

The 65 million plus long haulers worldwide have history to learn, skills to acquire, and knowledge to gain from those who have been living with chronic illness and disability for years. Crip doulas can offer the understanding and expertise that can only be acquired through experience.

In Conclusion: Disability Justice Beyond "Normal"

A final curious pandemic temporality to consider is the full-throated desire many evidence to return to "normal." Such a desire calls for an impossible movement back to something that never existed in the first place. Critical analysis of the conditions that sustain and neglect long COVID exposes the fabrication of any purported return to normal after the pandemic. But then again, normal never really existed. Perhaps the loss of the pre-pandemic normal is no loss at all, as disability rights activist Imani Barbarin (2022) suggests:

> "Normal" was a lie meant to pacify us and discourage challenging a society built around racism, ableism, and white supremacy… To want normal says that you have identified all of the issues put on display and said, "I'm fine with that." Unfortunately, the rest of us cannot be and never have been alright with normal. To move forward and change nothing despite what we have learned about these systemic failures and the people they affect would be a complete failure to protect ourselves from this happening again.

If long COVID accomplishes nothing else, it undoubtedly rips away the curtain to reveal a myriad of failures. These long COVID failures show us what most needs our collective moral attention and political focus now and into the future. The various ways in which disability justice scholars call for a reckoning with the complex interlocking set of injustices surrounding long COVID means that there can never be a return to normal. More importantly, there ought not be.

As public health experts remind us, the question is not if another pandemic will happen, but when. The imperative to refuse the push for a return to normal thus serves not only as a keen reminder of the ongoing injustices of long COVID we must address now but also underscores the necessity of meeting future pandemics and the post-infection syndromes they generate with heightened attention to justice and equitable care.

Notes

1 The Department of Health and Human Services defines Long COVID as: "a patient created term broadly defined as signs, symptoms, and conditions that continue or develop after initial SARS-CoV-2 infection. The signs, symptoms, and conditions are present four weeks or more after the initial phase of infection; may be multisystemic; and may present with a relapsing-remitting pattern and progression or worsen over time, with the possibility of severe and life-threatening events even months or years after infection. Long COVID is not one condition. It represents potentially overlapping entities, likely with different biological causes and different sets of risk factors and outcomes" (Department of Health and Human Services 2024).
2 The study Mulcahy references is Costa, et al. 2022.
3 It is important to note that a March 2024 letter to the *Lancet* questions the methodology used to determine the estimation of prevalence in the March 2023 editorial. Szanyi, Howe, and Blakely (2024) write: "the assertion that 65 million people worldwide had long COVID in March 2023, originated from a narrative review published in the same month. To arrive at this figure, the authors ostensibly took an estimate of symptom prevalence 90–150 days after SARS-CoV-2 infection from a single pre-omicron study conducted in the Netherlands of largely unvaccinated adults and then applied this estimate to the cumulative number of reported COVID-19 cases globally to date. This method is invalid. For example, this estimate assumed that long COVID never resolves and ignored studies indicating that vaccination reduces risk of long COVID by approximately 50%. Additionally, differences by SARS-CoV-2 variant were not considered, despite evidence showing up to a 75% reduction in long COVID occurrence among omicron (B.1.1.529) infections compared with delta variant infections" (1136–1137).
4 The complete list of "The Ten Principles of Disability Justice" contains the following: Intersectionality; Leadership of Those Most Impacted; Anti-Capitalist Politic; Cross-Movement Solidarity; Recognizing Wholeness; Sustainability; Commitment to Cross-Disability Solidarity; Interdependence; Collective Access; Collective Liberation.
5 Note that the fourth principle is referred to as Cross-Movement Solidarity in Berne et al. 2018 and as Commitment to Cross-Movement Organizing on the Sins Invalid 2015.

Work Cited

Barbarin, Imani. 2022. "You're Never Getting 'Normal' Back." *Crutches & Spice*, February 11, 2022. https://crutchesandspice.com/2022/02/11/%EF%BF%BCyoure-never-getting-normal-back/

Berne, Patricia, Aurora Levins Morales, David Langstaff and Invalid Sins. 2018. "Ten Principles of Disability Justice." *Women's Studies Quarterly* 46 (1/2): 227–230.

Bull-Otterson, Lara, Sarah Baca, Sharon Saydah, Tegan K. Boehmer, Stacey Adjei, Simone Gray, and Aaron M. Harris. 2022. "Post-COVID Conditions Among Adult COVID-19 Survivors Aged 18–64 and ≥65 Years — United States, March 2022–November 2021." *Morbidity and Mortality Weekly Report* 71 (21): 713–717.

Burns, Alice. 2024. "As Recommendations for Isolation End, How Common is Long COVID?" *KFF*, April 9, 2024. https://www.kff.org/coronavirus-covid-19/issue-brief/as-recommendations-for-isolation-end-how-common-is-long-covid/

Choutka, Jan, Viraj Jansari, Mady Hornig, and Akiko Iwasaki. 2022. "Unexplained Post-Acute Infection Syndromes." *Nature Medicine* 28: 911–923.

Clare, Eli. 2017. *Brilliant Imperfection: Grappling with Cure*. Durham: Duke University Press.

Costa, Bruno Almeida, Kaiza Vilarinho da Luz, Sarah Emanuelle Viana Campos, Germison Silva Lopes, João Paulo de Vasconcelos Leitão, and Fernando Barroso Duartea. 2022. "Can SARS-CoV-2 Induce Hematologic Malignancies in Predisposed Individuals? A Case Series and Review of the Literature." *Hematology, Transfusion and Cell Therapy* 44 (1): 26–31.

Cox, Tracy. 2021. "How Many People get 'Long COVID'? More Than Half, Researchers Find." *Penn State University*, October 21, 2021. https://www.psu.edu/news/research/story/how-many-people-get-long-covid-more-half-researchers-find/

Department of Health and Human Services. 2024. "Terms and Definitions." March 26, 2024. https://www.covid.gov/be-informed/longcovid/about#term

Ducharme, Jamie. 2022. "At Least 20% of People Who Get COVID-19 Develop Lingering Conditions, CDC Study Says." *Time Magazine*, May 25, 2022. https://time.com/6180861/covid-19-health-problems-after-recovery/

Faghy, Mark A, Rebecca Owen, Callum Thomas, James Yates, Francesco V. Ferraro, Lindsay Skipper, Sarah Barley-McMullen, Darren A Brown, Ross Arena, and Ruth E.M. Ashton. 2022. "Is Long COVID the Next Global Health Crisis?" *Journal of Global Health* 12 (2022): 1–6.

Groff, Destin, Ashley Sun, Anna E. Ssentongo, Djibril M. Ba, Nicholas Parsons, Govinda R. Poudel, Alain Lekoubou, John S. Oh, Jessica E. Ericson, Paddy Ssentongo, Vernon M. Chinchilli. 2021. "Short-term and Long-term Rates of Postacute Sequelae of SARS-CoV-2 Infection: A Systematic Review." *JAMA Network Open* 4 (10): 1–17.

Hannah E. Davis, Lisa McCorkell, Julia Moore Vogel and Eric J. Topol. 2023. "Long COVID: Major Findings, Mechanisms and Recommendations." *Nature Reviews Microbiology* 21: 133–146.

Khullar, Dhruv, Yongkang Zhang, Chengxi Zang, Zhenxing Xu, Fei Wang, Mark G. Weiner, Thomas W. Carton, Russell L. Rothman, Jason P. Block, Rainu Kaushal. 2023. "Racial/Ethnic Disparities in Post-acute Sequelae of SARS-CoV-2 Infection in New York: An EHR-Based Cohort Study from the RECOVER Program." *Journal of General Internal Medicine* 38 (5): 1127–1136.

Lancet. 2023. "Long COVID: 3 Years In," *The Lancet* 401 (10379): 795.

Long COVID Justice Project. n.d. "Pandemics Are Chronic: A Statement of Commitment to Long COVID Justice." *Long COVID Justice*. https://longcovidjustice.org/pandemics-are-chronic/

Lowe, Derek. 2022. "Long COVID, Long Other Things." *Science*, June 9, 2022. https://www.science.org/content/blog-post/long-covid-long-other-things

Mazer, Benjamin. 2022. "Long COVID Could Be a 'Mass Deterioration Event'." *The Atlantic*, June 15, 2022. https://www.theatlantic.com/health/archive/2022/06/long-covid-chronic-illness-disability/661285/

Mingus, Mia. 2022. "You Are Not Entitled to Our Deaths: COVID, Abled Supremacy & Interdependence." *Leaving Evidence*, January 16, 2022. https://leavingevidence.wordpress.com/2022/01/16/you-are-not-entitled-to-our-deaths-covid-abled-supremacy-interdependence/

Mulcahy, Lisa. 2023. "COVID and Leukemia: What's the Connection?" *WebMD.com*, May 31, 2023. https://www.webmd.com/covid/news/20230531/covid-and-leukemia-whats-the-connection

National Center for Health Statistics. "Long COVID Household Pulse Survey." *National Center for Health Statistics*, May 18, 2023. https://www.cdc.gov/nchs/covid19/pulse/long-covid.htm

Ndugga, Nambi, Latoya Hill, and Samantha Artiga. 2022. "COVID-19 Cases and Deaths, Vaccinations, and Treatments by Race/Ethnicity as of Fall 2022." *KFF*, November 17, 2022. https://www.kff.org/racial-equity-and-health-policy/issue-brief/covid-19-cases-and-deaths-vaccinations-and-treatments-by-race-ethnicity-as-of-fall-2022/

"PASC Dashboard." *American Academy of Physical Medicine and Rehabilitation*. https://pascdashboard.aapmr.org/

Pfaff, Emily R., Charisse Madlock-Brown, John M. Baratta, Abhishek Bhatia, Hannah Davis, Andrew Girvin, Elaine Hill, Liz Kelly, Kristin Kostka, Johanna Loomba, Julie A. McMurry, Rachel Wong, Tellen D. Bennett, Richard Moffitt, Christopher G. Chute, Melissa Haendel, N3C Consortium, RECOVER Consortium. 2023. "Coding Long COVID: Characterizing a New Disease through an ICD-10 Lens." *BMC Medicine* 21 (1): 58.

Piepzna-Samarasinha, Leah Lakshmi. 2018. *Care Work: Dreaming Disability Justice*. Vancouver: Arsenal Pulp Press.

Piepzna-Samarasinha, Leah Lakshmi. 2022. *The Future Is Disabled: Prophecies, Love Notes and Mourning Songs*. Vancouver: Arsenal Pulp Press.

Puar, Jasbir. 2017. *The Right to Maim: Debility, Capacity, Disability*. Durham: Duke University Press
Schmidt, Charles. 2023. "Do Repeat COVID Infections Increase the Risk of Severe Disease or Log COVID?" *Scientific American*, February 15, 2023. https://www.scientificamerican.com/article/do-repeat-covid-infections-increase-the-risk-of-severe-disease-or-long-covid/
Sins Invalid. 2015. "10 Principles of Disability Justice." September 17, 2015. https://www.sinsinvalid.org/blog/10-principles-of-disability-justice
Szanyi, Joshua. Samantha Howe, and Tony Blakely. 2024. "The Importance of Reporting Accurate Estimates of Long COVID Prevalence." *The Lancet* 403 (10432): 1136–1137.
WebMD Editorial Contributors. 2022. "Coronavirus and COVID-19: What You Should Know." *WebMD*, December 26, 2022. https://www.webmd.com/covid/news/20220420/30-percent-of-covid-patients-in-study-developed-long-covid

9

NOT EVERYTHING IS A PANDEMIC

The Challenge of Disability Justice

Perry Zurn

We have lived in pandemic times. While SARS-CoV-1 first appeared in 2002—an outbreak that affected 29 countries and resulted in 774 deaths—SARS-CoV-2 surfaced in 2019 and has since produced a worldwide pandemic resulting in over 7 million reported deaths at the time of writing. For many, everyday life in the USA quickly reoriented around risk calculations, mask mandates, social distancing practices, and vaccination campaigns. Hospitals and urgent care centers were (and to this day remain) strained. The country experienced massive job loss, business closures, unprecedented inflation, and government aid, while especially white-collar work shifted increasingly to remote, digital, or hybrid models pocked by stints of isolation and quarantine. Rates of anxiety and depression, and suicidality among the young, grew. Few familial units remain untouched by COVID-related sickness and death, and roughly a quarter of early COVID cases resulted in "long COVID," which involves persistent symptoms due to viral damage of heart, brain, and/or lungs (Huang et al. 2021). COVID turned everyday life in the US upside down. To say we have lived in pandemic times, then, is to say that we have lived day in and day out in the shadow of COVID.

But we purportedly live in pandemic times for still other reasons. Our times are marked by many threats to public health. The past suite of years evince a thicket of xenophobia; anti-Asian hate; anti-transgender legislation and rising trans exclusionary radical feminist (TERF) rhetoric; anti-Black violence and resistance; the #MeToo Movement and higher rates of sexual and domestic violence; immigration crises; a steeply exacerbated wealth gap; relentless attacks on Indigenous resurgence; disability discrimination, especially in healthcare and education; further entrenchment of prestige bias and Ivy League dominance; and the growth of climate change beyond all reasonable measure. In fact, it is hard to think of a social inequity that has not spiked in severity and social awareness since COVID hit the scene. Tellingly, it is equally hard to name a social inequity that has not itself been named a "pandemic" during this time.

I find this fast replication of the term *pandemic* curious. By some form of "contagion," so to speak, the term has jumped quickly, relentlessly from host to host. Reference to the "other" pandemic or the "second" pandemic has been repeatedly applied, for example, to racism (especially anti-Black and anti-Asian racism), xenophobia, sexual violence against women,

DOI: 10.4324/9781003502623-13

domestic violence, ableism, transphobic violence, colonial violence, class inequity, etc. The application of the term *pandemic* to these longstanding currents of social violence and inequity suggests that they are all social diseases fast jeopardizing world health, that they are a plague and a scourge to whole peoples and regions, and that they require immediate, emergency attention. The hailing of a second pandemic (and it is always only a second, marking a certain inability to think coalitionally), moreover, has appeared in such mainstream venues as the CDC, HRC, NPR, UN, *Time Magazine*, *New York Times*, *Harvard Law*, *Brookings Institution*, *Forbes*, *Times Higher Education*, American Academy of Pediatrics, etc., not to mention everyday conversations on Facebook and Twitter.

Before evaluating whether this explosion in the use of the term *pandemic* is helpful or not and to what ends, I want to consider the conditions that make this secondary use of the term *pandemic* possible. In what follows, I investigate both the persuasiveness and the appropriateness of the term *pandemic* applied to social inequities and/or systems of social oppression. In applying the term *pandemic* in these ways, people appeal not only to urgency and crisis, but also to disease and illness. Why that appeal? Why here, why now? And what are its conceptual and social implications? At minimum, I aim to pose a caution: the term *pandemic* may be neither appropriate nor helpful in these cases. More ambitiously, I draw on resources in disability justice to argue that the term *pandemic* applied to social inequities is ultimately inappropriate and dangerous. I am interested, overall, in the effects of this discourse on what it is possible (and impossible) to think, and what is it possible (and impossible) to do.

A Contagious Term

Both contagion and contingency stem from the same Latin roots: *com* (with) and *tangere* (to touch). Something touched off, here; COVID touched a nerve. The breadth and rapidity of the application of *pandemic* to a variety of social inequities is astonishing. It is as if it could not be helped, whether because the temptation of an easy metaphor was too much to resist or because the similarities were too true not to highlight. Here, I document just a slice of the litany of such uses available for analysis, focusing in particular on sexual violence, anti-Asian racism, anti-Black racism, colonialism, economic disparity, anti-trans violence, and ableism. Throughout, it is not just the temporal coincidence or the shared spatial extensiveness of COVID and social inequities that fuel the association. Rather, each social issue finds in COVID a unique resonance. These distinctive resonances are the deeper conditions that make the attribution of the term *pandemic* to social inequities possible.[1]

Sexual Violence

When it comes to sexual violence, especially against women, the claim is clear. Just as COVID spreads silently, often with so little awareness that the true number of cases remains a mystery, so sexual violence spreads silently, devastatingly. Importantly, in the latter case, that silence is reinforced: survivors are told (directly and indirectly) to keep silent. The UN Women (n.d.) website currently features a report entitled, "The Shadow Pandemic: Violence Against Women During COVID." The page outlines the pandemic-related intensification of an already severe rate of physical and sexual violence against women, especially by intimate partners. The Harvard Medical School calls it "A Second, Silent Pandemic," marking the increasingly strained support systems (e.g., rape crisis centers, domestic violence shelters, and mental health clinics) for survivors of sexual and domestic violence (Walker 2020). And *Forbes* calls it "The Other Pandemic," emphasizing its rampant presence in wars around the globe (Ochab 2021). While highlighting this shared mode of silent spread, writers are also frustrated by the bombast COVID has garnered on the political stage in comparison to the minimal coverage of sexual violence.

Anti-Asian Racism

As COVID swept the US in 2020, then President Trump repeatedly referred to it as the "Chinese virus," ostensibly signaling its origin in Wuhan, China (Rogers, Jake, and Swanson 2020). In doing so, he fed an already existing prejudice that Asian people are not only virus-carriers, but that they are a virus themselves, infiltrating US borders, hijacking American jobs, etc. With an insistent defiance, Asian people and their allies flipped this message on its head. First, they created a social media meme, in which individuals photographed themselves holding a sign that read "I am not a virus"—which itself went viral. Second, they diagnosed anti-Asian hate as itself the viral "pandemic." As Rep. Grace Meng stated upon the passing of the COVID-19 Hate Crimes Act, in May 2021, the Asian-American community has had to face an "additional pandemic: the virus of hate and bigotry" (Spunt 2021).[2] As early as October 2020, Harvard Law's publication *Bill of Health* identified "xenophobia" as the "second" pandemic faced by Asian Americans (Mohapatra 2020; cf. Silva 2020 and Cheng and Conca-Cheng 2020). Even more presciently, in March 2020, *Time Magazine* published a piece that, in addressing anti-Asian hate, warned that unless our societies, like our immune systems, "rapidly learn to recognize and eliminate novel microbes," we will continue to suffer from pandemics of "fear, panic, and xenophobia" (Shah 2020). This rhetorical move is a clever application of tactical counterveillance: it reverses the pathologizing gaze (Welch 2011).

Anti-Black Racism

In the case of anti-Black racism, the appeal to the term pandemic typically coincides with references to existing health inequities (only exacerbated by COVID) which contribute to slow death within Black communities. Slow death refers to the enervation in the microfibers of everyday life traceable to structural oppression, often naming the health costs of precarity and discrimination, trauma, and inherited trauma (Zurn 2019a). That slow death, moreover, is not wholly unlike weeks on a respirator, in a medically induced coma, before someone pulls the plug: it is a halflife, a suspended temporality. Of course, it is impossible to think COVID and anti-Black racism without also hearing the resonance between respiratory distress and George Floyd's repeated plea, "I can't breathe." In 2021, the CDC Director Rochelle Walensky named racism an "epidemic" in the US. Medical journals have gone one step farther, referring to anti-Black racism as not only "the other pandemic" (Godlee, 2020) but also "a pandemic on a pandemic" (Laurencin and Walker 2020). In the field of education, *Education Week* has referred to it as a "400-year-old pandemic" (Hutchings, Jr. 2021). Both *Education Week* and *Times Higher Education* (McCoy and Lee 2021) refer to the coincidence of COVID and anti-Black racism as a "dual pandemic." In *Chatelaine*, the leading women's magazine in Canada, Bee Quammie (2020) writes, "Racism—the cause of so much illness, anxiety, and death—is the pandemic that Black people live under all of our lives. [...] The pandemic of anti-Black racism has ravaged this country and the entire world for centuries—this is our time to eradicate it, to create a 'new normal' that is healthy for us all."

Colonialism

Colonialism spreads; it is inherently a spreading thing, and it ravages whole peoples and lands. In April 2020, Indigenous Action released, as part of its "art of resistance" series, a poster that reads: "Capitalism is a virus; colonialism is a plague" (Indigenous Action 2020). While scientifically, a plague is bacterial in nature (rather than viral), colloquially a plague refers to any infectious disease; as such, the poster presents capitalism and colonialism as interconnected threats. The poster's central image is a chemical warfare mask with two feathers sticking out of the top; the reference to breath is searing. As Greta Gaard wrote in June 2020, "the pandemic of colonialism [...] decimated Indigenous communities, deforested entire regions, pushed alcohol consumption, provided blankets with smallpox virus, entwined conquest with sexual violence against women and children, shot wolves and bison to near-extinction, and extracted oil, uranium, and coal from native lands while 'relocating' Indigenous survivors to underfunded 'reservations.'" This pandemic, moreover, is not simply in the past. University of Toronto Medicine recently bemoaned "the deadly pandemic of Anti-Indigenous Racism in healthcare" today (Department of Family and Community Medicine 2020). Appealing to the intimacies that subtend both the virus and Indigenous resurgence, Gaard concludes, "Only in the present might we breathe—and possibly be infected by the coronavirus. Or we can breathe in the awareness of our interbeing and align our behaviors accordingly" (Gaard 2020). It is through biohuman intimacies that colonialism can be resisted.

Economic Disparity

The steep climbs of COVID cases and deaths developed along equally steep climbs of wealth among the wealthiest few, and the steep losses of small businesses and the poor. The *London News* refers to the "two pandemic story" of COVID and "pandemic class inequality" (Lyon 2021). The Brookings Institution similarly refers to the economic "inequality pandemic" (Qureshi 2020). Brookings author Qureshi marks that because the COVID pandemic has privileged the digital economy, and hit low-skill, low-wage work the hardest, its costs "are borne disproportionately by poorer segments of society" and the world. This is exacerbated further by the soaring endowments of prestige schools and their steady, if not growing, applicant pools (Jaschik 2021). The rich do indeed get richer.

Anti-Trans Violence

Epidemics affect one population, while pandemics stretch across countries or continents. Despite glaring evidence to the contrary, anti-trans violence has for years—at least since 2014—been referred to in the US as an "epidemic" (Lorenz 2015 and Zigo 2017; Stankorb 2014). The HRC has relentlessly underscored this categorization (HRC 2018, 2021).[3] However, anti-trans violence, which includes bullying and abuse, physical assault, sexual assault, domestic violence, and murder, has recently graduated to "pandemic" status. This is not because people finally recognized the variety of assaults to bodily integrity (including injury, torture, and killing) that mark a global response to trans and gender non-conforming people. Rather, in cases where the shift in nomenclature is more than an upgrade in urgency, it is due to the "outbreak" of TERF rhetoric in the UK (via the likes of JK Rowling and Kathleen Stock) and its reverberations around the globe. Recognizing the power of rhetoric to fuel hate, anti-trans violence has now been called a "pandemic" (Mollmann 2021).[4] The contagion of words made it possible to think the spread of deeds.

Ableism

The metaphor of the pandemic is so rhetorically powerful that it appears to be applied to whatever problem is at hand. In this context, ableism, too, has been called a "pandemic." Ableism is the "virus you forgot to panic for," writes Connie Chen, in *The Harvard Crimson*, a virus that has met with widespread "indifference" and for which "no scientist is working on the cure" (2020). Having reached pandemic proportions, Chen argues, the virus of ableism must be eradicated. In her recent prayer, Rabbi Nikki DeBlosi (2020) invokes a world in which such eradication involves building "new institutions that refuse to deem [God's] creatures disposable." Sounding a similar note, Rabbi Elliot Kukla (2021), in a piece for the *New York Times*, insists, "#NoBodyIsDisposable." Posing the haunting question "Where is the vaccine for ableism?", Kukla highlights the relative "state-sanctioned callousness" that marks the US response to disability. Interestingly, much like Greta Gaard, Kukla finds in breath both danger and promise. "Viruses flourish," he writes, "each breath we exhale could be someone else's inhalation;" the vaccine for ableism might lie precisely here, in embracing rather than disavowing our intimacies and interdependence (2021). There is a certain irony, of course, in thinking ableism as a virus while the COVID virus disables large swaths of the population. US Department of Health and Human Services announced in 2021 that, in cases where long COVID is a "physical or mental impairment" that "can substantially limit one or more major life activities," it warrants ADA accommodation (Department of Health and Human Services [HHS] 2021). Millions of Americans are projected to be swept up by the "tsunami of disability" COVID brings (Pomeroy 2021).

What a litany. In retrospect, the term *pandemic* has been applied in recent years to many—if not most—of the major social inequities in US discourse. And it has been applied not only in everyday social media platforms such as Facebook and Twitter but also in high-level media outlets, indicating a deep cultural embrace of the nomenclature. This is no real surprise. That COVID is silent, that it spreads, that it suffocates, that its extent and severity continually go unrecognized, that it targets already marginalized populations with a heavier burden—all of these are good reasons that the COVID pandemic fast became a metaphor for social ills of all sorts, which are themselves silently spreading, suffocating, and yet underappreciated. It makes sense as a tactic to capitalize on these resonances, but, as I now turn to argue, there are other resonances that should make us pause and re-evaluate the tactic.

Making Sense, Not Making Sense

Having observed the fact that the term *pandemic* has spread to multiple continents of social concern and suggested some of the resonances that explain transmissibility in each case, I want to pause to assess more directly why the use of the term does and does not make sense. My aim is to pose a caution, to insist that the application of the term *pandemic* to social inequities is perhaps as troubling as it is easy. This is not to say that there are not other vantage points from which to analyze this conjunction. There is, for example, a wonderful invitation to think about the aerosolized particulates that subtend the transmissibility of COVID and the corollary words embedding in social airways that sediment the social inequities of racism, sexism, ableism, classism, colonialism, etc. A recuperative analysis of the association, however, is not my aim here. My aim is to pause and post a warning.

Making sense, of course, is dependent upon a set of contingent criteria that are internal to a given socio-linguistic system. When I say, then, that the application of the term *pandemic* to social inequities—at the height of the COVID pandemic and across a volatile political land-scape—makes sense, I grant the localism of this claim: it makes sense with respect to both the moment and the social movements in which it occurs. I want to read this shift in terminology first with a hermeneutic of charity, before turning to critique. For Willard Quine (2013) or Donald Davidson (1973), a hermeneutic of charity involves maximizing the truth or rational-ity of a claim. Still more deeply, it involves reading, á la María Lugones (2003a), with loving perception, trying to understand a claim on its own terms and traveling to each other's "worlds of sense" (80).

Here, then, are five major reasons why the terminological shift admittedly makes sense, even if, as I will show, the shift is ultimately unsustainable and unjustifiable.

1 *Contiguous Crises*: It makes sense, tactically, to capitalize on the exigency of a term—and of a moment—in order to get other concerns heard. Appealing to one crisis, especially when that crisis is ongoing, to get another crisis recognized is strategic. Applying the term *pandemic* to social inequities during the COVID pandemic is, then, just such a strategy and tactic. Stemming from the Greek *krinein*, meaning "to decide," the word *crisis* connotes a moment of decision, a decisive turning point, in which fate turns toward life or toward death. Coinciding with repeated appeals to flatten the COVID curve or quell the surge have been repeated calls for accountability and reckoning with longstanding histories of social violence and social death along any number of identitarian axes. Linking these shared urgencies through the term *pandemic* makes strategic sense. Perhaps if the crises are equally felt, there may be a shared turning point.

2 *Collective Responsibility*: It makes sense because, just as everyone is expected to do their part in addressing COVID (e.g., mask, social distance, get vaccinated and boosted, quar-antine, etc.), so everyone must do their part to address social inequities. The latter requires a commitment to act responsibly in a variety of ways, including but not limited to educat-ing oneself, building new habits of speech and action, practicing allyship, and organizing change. The call to collective action is, of course, wholly justified in each case. Just as we cannot be an agglomeration of alienated monadic entities in an effective front against COVID, the same is true if we are to build capacity to resist and dismantle social inequities (Young 1990). Putting the widespread insistence on collective responsibility for COVID in the service of social inequities by applying the term *pandemic* promises to increase the lat-ter's traction in public discourse.

3 *Unique Resonances*: It makes sense because working and thinking in pandemic times has unearthed certain instructive resonances between COVID and specific social inequities that would otherwise go unnoticed. This is the insight of coincidence, but it is insight none-theless. And that insight is irrevocably local insofar as it regards not simply pandemics in general but COVID in particular, and not simply social inequity writ large but the social inequities that fire political imaginations of today. It takes remarkable attentiveness and ingenuity to draw out the shared modes of silence, spreading, respiratory distress, suffoca-tion, social death, health inequity, steep climbs and big gaps, indifference, callousness, and interdependence. These sonorities deserve a hearing.

4 *Public Health Crises*: It makes sense because social inequities do produce health inequali-ties and, in some cases, public health crises. It is, then, a short rhetorical step, during pan-demic times, from "public health crisis" to "pandemic" (Beech et al. 2021). A pandemic matters, after all, because it threatens the health of the world population. When social

inequities, and the systems of oppression undergirding them, compromise not only the health and safety, but the well-being and capacity to flourish of large swaths of specific demographics across borders and boundaries, "pandemic" seems like a reasonable, if not a necessary, categorization.

5 *Interlocking Inequities*: It makes sense because the causal intimacies between COVID and social inequities are deep and often unseen. The COVID pandemic exacerbates social inequities, driving the poor into greater poverty and subjecting those marginalized by race, disability, or gender non-conformity into greater health precarity. Just as surely, social inequities exacerbate the COVID pandemic, surging through low-income communities, communities of color, and Indigenous communities. The two are intertwined and intersecting, and that is important not only to recognize but to insist upon as ameliorative policy and health recommendations get underway. The exigency, then, of thinking two pandemics, or a pandemic within a pandemic, or a pandemic on a pandemic, helps conceptualize these forces caught egging one another on in an apparent death spiral.

Not everything about this new application of the term *pandemic* makes sense, however. As I turn, now, from a hermeneutic of charity to a hermeneutic of suspicion, I want to ask: What might not be right about this formulation? Why might it be unhelpful, at least, and even harmful, at most? As defined by Paul Ricoeur (2008), the hermeneutic of suspicion involves getting behind the text in order to secure its deeper meaning and hidden sense. I am less interested in getting behind than in getting underneath. Drawing on the sense of suspicion utilized in critical theory, from Max Horkheimer (2002) to Michel Foucault (1997) and Judith Butler (2004, 2009), I want to ask: What is at work here that might otherwise go unnoticed? What sleights of hand are in play? What ideological and institutional complicities subtend the turn? And what concerning social implications follow?

Here are five major reasons why the terminological shift of applying *pandemic* to social inequities does not make sense.

1 *Disaster Capitalism*: It does not make sense so much as it makes capital. When a specific way of framing a problem gains cultural currency, it garners widespread (and widespreading) endorsement due to the clout of its claimants. The clout of claimants, however, is never a good reason for endorsement and is in fact a great reason to pause and re-evaluate the claim. The CDC, HRC, NPR, UN, *Time Magazine*, *New York Times*, *Harvard Law*, *Brookings Institution*, *Forbes*, and *Times Higher Education* all think the application of *pandemic* to social inequities makes sense. Why might these public and academic heavyweights have found this formulation comparatively easy to swallow, hook-line-and-sinker? And what might that formulation therefore be doing (and not doing) for them? Arguably, the pronouncement of not one but *two* pandemics participates in a form of disaster capitalism that retroactively casts said institutions as cutting-edge culture warriors whose incisive voice in multiple crises deserves respect, media following, and organizational funding (Klein 2008). Such deployments of shocking social assessments and commensurate virtue signaling, moreover, typically mask a complicity with ongoing trajectories of social inequities, as well as an inability to address (or a tractable indifference toward) the issues themselves.

2 *Technical Term*: It does not make sense because, technically, pandemics are pandemics and social inequities are social inequities. Not to get too exacting here, but a pandemic is an infectious disease that affects people across populations while social inequities are

structural hierarchies that are rooted in systems of oppression. Even if one were to use *pandemic* as a persuasive metaphor, its structure is not appropriate. A pandemic is a disease that manifests as a quickly uncontrolled outbreak that spreads from one source point to multiple hubs across countries and/or continents. It strikes suddenly and sweeps through devastatingly. Pandemic time, here, is critical to its function. By contrast, racism, sexual violence, and ableism, for example, are centuries, even millennia in the making. They appear to be endemic to the globe. A better immunological metaphor for them, then, might be a chronic autoimmune disease, that through which the (social) body attacks itself.

3 *Naturalized Threat*: It does not make sense because the application of *pandemic* to social inequities inaccurately (and unhelpfully) indicates that people "catch" the contagious virus of racism, colonialism, ableism, misogyny, transphobia, or wealth inequity. In doing so, the move naturalizes the threat rather than historicizes the threat, and it subjectivizes the response. If social inequities are traceable to contagious behaviors and attitudes, contracted through individual interactions, rather than to social structures sedimented within a wide variety of institutions, then the call is to stay healthy and not catch these social ills as they make their rounds. While it is true that we acquire racist, colonial, ableist, misogynist, transphobic, and classist habits of thought and deed through social interaction, this has been better theorized as an inheritance linked to history rather than a contagion confined to the immediate present. In the latter theorization, we are already saturated by these investments of socially oppressive systems and dismantling them then becomes a transhistorical rather than reactive project.

4 *State Response*: It does not make sense, as a strategy for progressive politics, because, in addition to subjectivizing the response, it centralizes the response. Conceptualizing social inequities as pandemics implicitly invokes biopolitical redress. The best line of defense against a pandemic is state-sanctioned policies and protocols implemented at the national and international levels. The top-down strategy ensures, ultimately, that the disease is controlled or suppressed. This invocation, however, on the part of social justice advocates, worryingly de-emphasizes personal responsibility, local organizing, mutual aid projects, and nonstate/anti-state resistance strategies and their long histories (Spade 2020). Calling for (state-generated and state-distributed) vaccines for racism, colonialism, ableism, misogyny, transphobia, classism, and wealth gaps is, arguably, like appealing to administratively initiated DEI policies that replace and often frustrate the more difficult, but more effective work of supporting local marginalized communities in their own organizing efforts and collective flourishing (Ahmed 2012). What gets centralized in the response matters.

5 *Call for Cure*: It does not make sense, again as a strategy of progressive politics, because, in calling social inequities "pandemics," the turn appeals to the ideal of a "healthy" social body and sounds the call for a "cure" (Clare 2017). It capitalizes on public fear of disease in general. This trope of protecting the health of the social body by suppressing all manner of moral ills and physical deformities has, for centuries, fueled ableist and eugenicist practices. It denies that living with illness, and living with the fact of moral failure, may in fact be the better part of social healing. For me, this fifth and final reason is the most important. This is the disability justice challenge, which I turn to develop in the final section.

I am not saying that describing the "pandemic" of ableism or sexual violence, for example, is complete and utter non-sense. I understand and appreciate its sources of sense. But I am saying that it does not make technical sense, nor does it make political sense for progressive movements. More specifically, there are layers of its sense-making that are deeply troubling. Its complicity in disaster capitalism, its insistence on state-sponsored redress, as well as the naturalization and pathologization of social ills all enervate the deeper work of collective social transformation. I understand, of course, that its use is merely tactical. However, if, as a biproduct of a useful association, we shore up neoliberal institutions and underscore one of the longest standing prejudices to have fueled major social inequities—i.e., that the health of the social body requires suppression of moral and physical pathologies—then we ultimately neutralize our tactic. Or, worse yet, we smuggle in, Trojan horse style, the very grounds of our work's own undoing. And that force of undoing may well outlive any advances we gain in the present.

A Disability Justice Challenge

What happens when we talk about racism as an uncontrolled disease rather than as a political system of oppression? When we call white supremacy a "plague" (Benjamin 2022, 39)? What happens when we apply pandemic terminology to ableism or rape? What gets thought and unthought when we mention viral surges in wealth inequity or transphobic violence, or when we underscore the contagion of colonialism? If social inequities are viral pathogens of this sort, the call is to eradicate them so as either to retain or to return to a healthy social body. The disease must be quelled and people must be cured. As Haley Jackson Manley (2020) of Baylor College of Medicine puts it, racism is "a disease that we must destroy the root of in order to find a cure." Subtending this call is a claim to the necessity of cure from illness as a moral and practical exigency. The claim replicates an old and dangerous habit of thought that has fueled puritanical and eugenic projects for centuries. For example, and put more directly, calling racism a disease mobilizes anti-disability sentiments and uses them to enhance the call to racial justice. At its heart, the move communicates sentiments of fear and disgust: To catch a soul-disfiguring virus, to be a disease-ridden social body, to individually manifest human dysfunction is a terrible thing. Such a life, whether individual or social, is simply not worth living (Reynolds 2022). Health must be sought quickly and aggressively.

Disability justice poses a fundamental challenge to this framework. In contrast with disability rights work that typically privileges single-issue analysis and accessibility solutions, disability justice demands an ongoing, perpetually abolitionist stance toward ableism (as part and parcel of multiple structures of oppression) through collective struggle and radical imagination (Sins Invalid 2020; Piepzna-Samarasinha 2022).[5] Disability justice is not here to win something; it is here to do the slow, real work of transformation. In the context of pandemic-related rhetoric, disability justice resists appeals to purity and to cure and refuses their underlying attachments to the ideal of health. Disability justice instead enjoins us to reckon with the inescapable impurities and illnesses of our bodies; the violence of cure in its appeal to a prior or future healthy (or "normal") body; and the interdependence required to live with varying needs and capacities. By fueling fear and disgust in relation to social inequities *by analogizing them to physical illness*, and specifically to the often disabling illness of COVID, the appeal to "pandemic" terminology across social justice movements fails to engage in deep coalitional thought and work.

Consider first the appeal to purity. As Alexis Shotwell (2016) details in her book *Against Purity*, the appeal to the natural body (unmarred by illness, injury, disease, and toxicity) and its concomitant appeal to moral purity (unmarked by complicity and entanglement) are keystones of ableist thinking. Insofar as they appeal to a present, past, or future in which "naturality" and "purity" are achieved and/or achievable, they are predicated on illusions—mere smoke and vapors. It is for this reason that Shotwell proposes an ethics of impurity. "All there is, while things perpetually fall apart, is the possibility of acting from where we are," she writes (4–5). What does it mean to deal with, live with, thrive with the fact that death, disease, illness, impairment, and toxicity happen? Purity is not only an ableist mindset, moreover; it is also a colonial and cisnormative mindset. María Lugones (2003b) argues that the politics of purity, predicated as it is on a logic of cleanliness and separation, is a colonial structure of control and isolation. Likewise, the politics of purity has repeatedly been used to hound and eradicate gender non-conformity from social life (Zurn 2019b). Indeed, hygienic regimes police and control the always unwieldy ambiguity that inescapably marks people on the social margins.

Consider second the appeal to a cure. Whether invoking spiritual salvation or medical correction, the ideology of cure has long marshalled a sustained attack on disability communities and posed an obstacle to disability justice. In their work, both Eli Clare (2017) and Eunjung Kim (2017) wrestle with the violent histories of cure. Cure, Kim argues, often involves a "violence that disfigures disability" (226). Cleverly reversing the longstanding conceptualization of disability as a disfigurement, Kim here describes the disfiguring *of* disability as not only a physical process but also a metaphysical one. It involves, she explains, "deny[ing] [disability's] aesthetic and ethical presence" by forcing the disabled body "to approximate the normal body" (226). This move, at the most basic level, "fail[s] to imagine the uncured body as a mode of being," imagining that body instead as not-being or as being-less (228). Clare similarly assumes a largely "anti-cure" stance. As he explains it, "cure requires damage" (15); which is to say, cure assumes that certain bodyminds are "defective," "undesirable," and "disposable" unless or until they are cured (23). Neither Kim, nor Clare, however, deny the fact that some members of the disability community desire and secure treatment. Supporting that collective multiplicity (in contrast to purity), Kim and Clare affirm medical treatment as an individual choice but critique the wholesale social expectation of cure—its language, histories, and practices.

Being against applying the term *pandemic* to sexual violence or racism or ableism does not mean being pro- sexual violence or racism or ableism. It means judging that the resonances and implications such an application mobilizes are counter to the work of liberation. I am not arguing that social inequities, *as social ills*, ought to be valued and celebrated in the way people with disabilities ought to be valued and celebrated in a society. I am saying that social inequities are best not referred to or understood as *social ills* in the first place. Mobilizing affect and action by calling social inequities and systems of oppression "pandemics" inadvertently but perniciously replicates cornerstones of ableist thinking: marshalling social amelioration through appeals to purity and cure. Given this issue, some might argue that we ought simply to rely on more accurate and literal assessments of structural violence. Metaphor, however, is not the problem here. Rather, critical awareness of which metaphors are being used, to what ends and with what effects, and accountability for what they call up or smuggle in, is crucial. When subjected to that kind of scrutiny, the metaphor of "pandemic" applied to social inequities does more harm than good.

I am also suggesting that there may be no pure social body to be had or to be dreamed. Moral failures are a real part of human social existence. With Kate Norlock (2019), I too think our movements are better served not by narratives that pose some final resolution (e.g., world peace, vaccines for ableism, etc.) but rather by narratives of praxis-centered ethics for "perpetual struggle." While Norlock's argument relies on the supposition that ending evil is an unjustifiable hope, I would argue that the goal of having gotten it right, having seen everything through, and having no more need to learn or grow is in fact a puritanical rather than a liberatory dream. The injunction then is to learn how to live in our nonideal world meaningfully—and transformatively—without narratives of victory or vanquishment, and without appealing to purity and to cure. To do so, several core principles of disability justice need to guide the way.

First, we will need coalitional work. Troublingly, the applications of *pandemic* to social inequities repeatedly appeal to single-axis resistance. The application seems to only ever invoke a "second" pandemic, the "shadow" pandemic, the "other" pandemic, "another" pandemic; or it refers to "two pandemics" or "dual pandemics," or to "the pandemic within a pandemic" or "a pandemic on a pandemic." These invocations obscure the very real fact that multiple social inequities, not to mention intersecting social inequities, structure society today. They also fail to honor the long and varied lineage of coalitional resistance (as if we have learned nothing from Gloria Anzaldúa, Patricia Hill Collins, bell hooks, Audre Lorde, etc.). They furthermore disavow complicity, as if one could test "positive" or "negative" in relation to the social virus, being either a spreader or an innocent bystander. This framework leaves no room for recognizing, let alone addressing, the way social inequities haunt and exacerbate one another, as much as the way marginalized communities retain a variety of systemic oppressions in their belly. Getting beyond binary code in the assessment of social inequities is crucial not only for capacity building between resistance movements but also for accountability work within them.

Second, we will need restorative and transformative justice work. There is a long and intimate connection between the curative and the carceral (cf. Ben-Moshe 2020). Across millennia, the repeated assessment of sickness as criminal and criminality as sick is hard to miss. That conjuncture, moreover, ensures that carceral and curative logics necessarily strengthen the circulation of violence in their names (Mingus 2019; Kaba 2021). Importantly, to capitalize on an ignorance/guilt model, solvable by policy and punishment, or to capitalize on the sick/healthy model, solvable by isolation, treatment, and cure, is to miss the crucial work of community building, restoration, and transformation (Massichis, Lee, and Spade 2011). It is one of the wisdoms of abolitionist literature that moral failures cannot be zapped by policy or police crackdowns or shuttled away into prisons. Moral failures permeate all human relations. Recognizing that fact, rather than disavowing it through appeals to cure and correction, is the foundation for healing and accountability practices. The aim of restorative and transformative justice work is not to correct human disease-bags, but to build ways of being with one another that reduce harm and strengthen community.

Third, we will need care work. Disability justice invokes a world not of carceral purity or medical cure, but of crip care. In Leah Lakshmi Piepzna-Samarasinha's *Care Work*, they describe care work as a "way of being," rather than as a crisis-centered state system (Piepzna-Samarasinha 2018). Care work, care webs, care-making, and care collectives, according to Piepzna-Samarasinha, are disability-led "experiments" in crip survival and flourishing that center the wholeness of people, the interdependence of people, and people's need for collective access. For Hil Malatino, writing at the jointure of crip and trans care, these are "forms of care that enable co-constituted, interdependent subjects to repair, rebuild, and cultivate resilience" (Malatino 2020, 43). The overall response to the COVID pandemic on the part of the disability community has been rich and varied. At the heart of that response is an injunction to center disabled people; reduce everyone's chances of contracting COVID (not just able-bodied people); and respect the non-standard quarantine and vaccination needs of those immuno-compromised or with co-morbidities. The community has also called for "crip doulas," to use Stacy Milburn's term, to help people newly disabled by long COVID find their way. This is an attitudinal shift toward positive care for and with those with neurodivergent minds, compromised bodies, and non-normative arrangements of health. Not to correct, or to cure, but to honor the "brokenbeautiful" (Gumbs). And it is in care worlds like these that the transformative work of dismantling systemic oppressions can best get underway.

The application of the term *pandemic* to social inequities is indeed too quick and too easy. While certain resonances, permitted by the application, are instructive and insightful, there are others that re-entrench histories and systems of ableism. The disability justice challenge is to re-orient attitudes and practices toward caring about vectors of disease and caring for those they affect. Care circles, within a disability justice framework, then build capacity to address systemic oppressions outside them, but also within.

* * *

I am all for utopian thinking. Thinking that inspires, that provides hope, that suggests more is possible. Thinking that equips us to struggle, against things outside us and within us, to uproot and to plant. Thinking for another world. But I am also for a thinking that is honest and that is humble. In her searing essay "The Pandemic is a Portal," Arundhati Roy (2020) beautifully invokes that other side:

> We can choose to walk through [the pandemic], dragging the carcasses of our prejudice and hatred, our avarice, our data banks and dead ideas, our dead rivers and smoky skies behind us. Or we can walk through lightly, with little luggage, ready to imagine another world. And ready to fight for it.

(132)

Let us indeed dream of a world in which our load of prejudices is lightened, and our bonds with hatred and avarice are broken in significant ways. But let us also dream of a world in which, whatever still clings to us and cannot be sloughed off (because of our failure to attain the fully willing, conscious, rational subjectivity the Enlightenment promised) is something we have the resources to address. Let us imagine, just as radically, that we bring with us the attunements necessary to critically navigate our existing and future complicities in social inequities. I dream not of a world without moral failures, but of a world in which we know what to do when we inevitably fail and are failed by one another.

Whatever success we may have in the present shifting attitudes and changing policies, whole social structures and histories lie in their wake, bearing down on our present and well into our futures. We cannot get outside of our histories; we can only ever work to transform them from within. And if that is our project, the metaphor of eradicating a pandemic of this or that social inequity is unhelpful at best.

Notes

1 While the use of metaphor is a basic cognitive tool, individual metaphors should be subject to critical investigation. See Lakoff and Johnson 2003 and Sontag 1978.
2 Cf. "The Epidemic of Anti-Asian Hate Must End," 2021.
3 Cf. "The Epidemic of Violence Against Transgender People," 202.
4 See also the common invective against the "pandemic" of anti-trans violence on Twitter.
5 See also Desiree Valentine's contribution to this volume.

Work Cited

Ahmed, Sara. 2012. *On Being Included: Racism and Diversity in Institutional Life*. Durham: Duke University Press.
Beech, Bettina M., Chandra Ford, Roland J. Thorpe Jr., Marino A. Bruce, and Keith C. Norris. 2021. "Poverty, Racism, and the Public Health Crisis in America." *Frontiers in Public Health*, September 6, 2021. https://www.frontiersin.org/articles/10.3389/fpubh.2021.699049/full
Ben-Moshe, Liat. 2020. *Decarcerating Disability: Deinstitutionalization and Prison Abolition*. Minneapolis: University of Minnesota Press.
Benjamin, Ruha. 2022. *Viral Justice: How We Grow the World We Want*. Princeton: Princeton University Press.
Butler, Judith. 2004. "What is Critique? An Essay on Foucault's Virtue." In *The Judith Butler Reader*, ed. Sara Salih, 302–322. Oxford: Wiley Blackwell.
Butler, Judith. 2009. "Critique, Dissent, Disciplinarity." *Critical Inquiry* 35 (4): 773–795.
Chen, Connie. 2020. "The Virus You Forgot to Panic For." *The Harvard Crimson*, April 16, 2020. https://www.thecrimson.com/article/2020/4/16/chen-virus-you-forgot-to-panic-for/
Cheng, Tina L. and Alison M. Conca-Cheng. 2020. "The Pandemics of Racism and COVID-19: Danger and Opportunity." *Pediatrics* 146 (5): e2020024836. https://doi.org/10.1542/peds.2020-024836
Clare, Eli. 2017. *Brilliant Imperfection: Grappling with Cure*. Durham: Duke University Press.
Davidson, Donald. 1973. "On the Very Idea of Conceptual Scheme." *Proceedings and Addresses of the American Philosophical Association* 47: 5–20.
Department of Family and Community Medicine. 2020. "Joyce Echaquan's Life Matters: Addressing the Deadly Pandemic of Anti-Indigenous Racism in Healthcare." *University of Toronto Medicine News*, October 9, 2020. https://dfcm.utoronto.ca/news/joyce-echaquans-life-matters-addressing-deadly-pandemic-anti-indigenous-racism-healthcare
Department of Health and Human Services. 2021. "Guidance on 'Long COVID' as a Disability under the ADA." *HHS.gov*, July 26, 2021. https://www.hhs.gov/civil-rights/for-providers/civil-rights-covid19/guidance-long-covid-disability/index.html
Foucault, Michel. 1997. "What is Critique?" In *The Politics of Truth*, ed. Sylvere Lotringer, 41–81. Los Angeles: Semiotext(e).
Gaard, Greta. 2020. "The Coronavirus as Messenger." *Bifrost Online*, June 8, 2020. https://bifrostonline.org/greta-gaard/
Godlee, Fiona. 2020. "Racism: The Other Pandemic." *British Medical Journal* 369: m2303. https://www.bmj.com/content/369/bmj.m2303
Horkheimer, Max. 2002. *Critical Theory: Selected Essays*, trans. Matthew J. O'Connell. New York: Continuum.
Huang, Yong, Melissa D. Pinto, Jessica L. Borelli, Milad Asgari Mehrabadi, Heather Abrihim, Nikil Dutt, Natalie Lambert, Erika L. Nurmi, Rana Shakraborty Amir M. Rahmani, and Charles A. Downs. 2021. "COVID Symptoms, Symptom Clusters and Predictors for Becoming a Long-Hauler: Looking for Clarity in the Haze of the Pandemic," *medRxiv*. https://doi.org/10.1101/2021.03.03.21252086
Human Rights Campaign. 2018. "A National Epidemic: Fatal Anti-Transgender Violence in America in 2018." *Human Rights Campaign*. https://www.hrc.org/resources/a-national-epidemic-fatal-anti-transgender-violence-in-america-in-2018
Human Rights Campaign. 2021. "An Epidemic of Violence 2021: Fatal Violence Against Transgender and Gender Non-Conforming People in the United States in 2021." *Human Rights Campaign*. https://reports.hrc.org/an-epidemic-of-violence-fatal-violence-against-transgender-and-gender-non-confirming-people-in-the-united-states-in-2021

Hutchings, Jr., Gregory C. 2021. "We Must Confront the Pandemic Within the Pandemic: Racism." *Education Week*, July 14, 2021. https://www.edweek.org/leadership/opinion-superintendent-pandemic-lesson-4-confront-the-pandemic-within-the-pandemic/2021/07

Indigenous Action. 2020. "Capitalism is a virus; colonialism is a plague." April 10, 2020. https://www.indigenousaction.org/capitalism-is-a-virus-colonialism-is-a-plague-poster/

Jaschik, Scott. 2021. "Admissions Have and Have-Nots." *Inside Higher Ed*, January 11, 2021. https://www.insidehighered.com/admissions/article/2021/01/11/admissions-cycle-favors-institutions-prestige-and-money

Kaba, Mariame. 2021. *We Do This 'Til We Free Us: Abolitionist Organizing and Transformative Justice*. New York: Haymarket Press.

Kim, Eunjung. 2017. *Curative Violence: Rehabilitating Disability, Gender, and Sexuality in Modern Korea*. Durham: Duke University Press.

Klein, Naomi. 2008. *The Shock Doctrine*. Toronto: Vintage.

Kukla, Elliot. 2021. "Where is the Vaccine for Ableism?" *New York Times*, February 4, 2021. https://www.nytimes.com/2021/02/04/opinion/covid-vaccine-ableism.html

Lakoff, George and Mark Johnson. 2003. *Metaphors We Live By*. Chicago: University of Chicago Press.

Laurencin, Cato T. and Joanne M. Walker. 2020. "A Pandemic on a Pandemic: Racism and COVID-19 in Blacks." *Cell Systems* 11: 9–10.

Lorenz, Brandon. 2015. "Human Rights Campaign Endorses Hilary Clinton for President." *Human Rights Campaign*, January 19, 2015. http://static.politico.com/52/c9/27180ecf41ae8383115f7fe0840e/hrc.pdf

Lugones, María. 2003a. "Playfulness and World-Traveling." In *Pilgrimages/Peregrinajes: Theorizing Coalition Against Multiple Oppressions*, 77–102. Lanham: Rowman and Littlefield.

Lugones, María. 2003b. "Purity, Impurity, and Separation." In *Pilgrimages/Peregrinajes: Theorizing Coalition Against Multiple Oppressions*, 121–150. Lanham: Rowman and Littlefield.

Lyon, Jason. 2021. "TUC calls for an economic reset to tackle pandemic class inequality." *London News Today*, September 9, 2021. https://londonnewstime.com/tuc-calls-for-an-economic-reset-to-tackle-pandemic-class-inequality/442295/

Malatino, Hil. 2020. *Trans Care*. Minneapolis: University of Minnesota Press.

Manley, Haley Jackson. 2020. "Racism: Not a Pandemic, but a Chronic Disease." *Baylor College of Medicine blog*, June 12, 2020. https://blogs.bcm.edu/2020/06/12/racism-not-a-pandemic-but-a-chronic-disease/

Massichis, Morgan, Alexander Lee, and Dean Spade. 2011. "Building an Abolitionist Trans and Queer movement with Everything We've Got." in *Captive Genders: Trans Embodiment and the Prison Industrial Complex*, eds. Eric Stanley and Nat Smith, 21–46. Chico: AK Press.

McCoy, Henrika and Madeline Y. Lee. 2021. "Minority Academics Face Dual Pandemics of COVID-19 and Racism." *Times Higher Education*, March 15, 2021. https://www.timeshighereducation.com/opinion/minority-academics-face-dual-pandemics-covid-19-and-racism

Mingus, Mia. 2019. "Transformative Justice: A Brief Description." *LeavingEvidence*, January 9, 2019. https://leavingevidence.wordpress.com/2019/01/09/transformative-justice-a-brief-description/

Mohapatra, Seema. 2020. "The Two Pandemics Facing Asian Americans: COVID-19 and Xenophobia." *Bill of Health*, October 1, 2020. https://blog.petrieflom.law.harvard.edu/2020/10/01/covid19-xenophobia-asian-americans/

Mollmann, Marianne. 2021. "Anti-Trans Rhetoric is Fueling a Pandemic of Violence." *The Fund for Global Human Rights*, December 2021. https://globalhumanrights.org/commentary/anti-trans-rhetoric-is-fueling-a-pandemic-of-violence/

Nikki, DeBlosi. 2020. "A Poem-Prayer Against Ableism." *Rabbinikki.medium.com*, March 26, 2020. https://rabbinikki.medium.com/a-poem-prayer-against-ableism-fbe16a61bdc0

Norlock, Kate. 2019. "Perpetual Struggle." *Hypatia* 34 (1): 6–19.

Ochab, Ewelina U. 2021. "The Other Pandemic: Rape and Sexual Violence in War." *Forbes Magazine*, June 14, 2021. https://www.forbes.com/sites/ewelinaochab/2021/06/14/the-other-pandemic-rape-and-sexual-violence-in-war/?sh=5456c0c43040

Piepzna-Samarasinha, Leah Lakshmi. 2018. *Care Work: Dreaming Disability Justice*. Vancouver: Arsenal Pulp Press.

Piepzna-Samarasinha, Leah Lakshmi. 2022. *The Future is Disabled: Prophecies, Love Notes, and Mourning Songs*. Vancouver: Aresenal Pulp Press.

Pomeroy, Claire. 2021. "A Tsunami of Disability is Coming as a Result of 'Long COVID'." *Scientific American*, July 6, 2021. https://www.scientificamerican.com/article/a-tsunami-of-disability-is-coming-as-a-result-of-lsquo-long-covid-rsquo/

Quammie, Bee. 2020. "Anti-Black Racism was Already a Pandemic." *Chatelaine*, June 10, 2020. https://www.chatelaine.com/living/anti-black-racism-pandemic/

Quine, W. V. O. 2013. *Word and Object*. Cambridge: MIT Press.

Qureshi, Zia. 2020. "Tackling the Inequality Pandemic: Is there a cure?" *Brookings Institution*, November 17, 2020. https://www.brookings.edu/research/tackling-the-inequality-pandemic-is-there-a-cure/

Reynolds, Joel Michael. 2022. *The Life Worth Living*. Minneapolis: University of Minnesota Press.

Ricoeur, Paul. 2008. *Freud and Philosophy*. New Haven: Yale University Press.

Rogers, Katie, Lara Jakes, and Ana Swanson. 2020. "Trump Defends Using 'Chinese Virus' Label, Ignoring Growing Criticism." *New York Times*, March 18, 2020. https://www.nytimes.com/2020/03/18/us/politics/china-virus.html

Roy, Arundhati. 2020. "The Pandemic Is a Portal." In *Azadi: Freedom. Fascism. Fiction*. New York: Haymarket Books.

Shah, Sonia. 2020. "The Pandemic of Xenophobia and Scapegoating." *TIME Magazine*, March 7, 2020. https://time.com/5776279/pandemic-xenophobia-scapegoating/

Shotwell, Alexis. 2016. *Against Purity: Living Ethically in Compromised Times*. Minneapolis: University of Minnesota Press.

Silva, H. M. 2020. "The Xenophobia Virus and the COVID-19 Pandemic." *Ethique & Santé* 18 (2): 102–106.

Sins Invalid. 2020. "What is Disability Justice?" June 16, 2020. https://www.sinsinvalid.org/news-1/2020/6/16/what-is-disability-justice

Sontag, Susan. 1978. *Illness as Metaphor*. New York: Farrar, Straus, & Giroux.

Spade, Dean. 2020. *Mutual Aid: Building Solidarity During this Crisis (and the Next)*. New York: Verso.

Spunt, Barbara. 2021. "Congress Passes Bill to Combat 'Second Pandemic' of Anti-Asian Hate." *KQED*, May 18, 2021. https://www.kqed.org/news/11874204/congress-passes-bill-to-combat-second-pandemic-of-anti-asian-hate

Stankorb, Sarah. 2014. "The Unsteady Shelf Life of a Social Justice Symbol." *Good*, October 15, 2014. https://www.good.is/features/cece-mcdonald-social-movement

"The epidemic of anti-Asian hate must end." 2021. *Lighthouse.lyndhurstschools.net*, May 26, 2021. http://lighthouse.lyndhurstschools.net/2021/05/26/the-epidemic-of-anti-asian-hate-must-end/

"The Epidemic of Violence Against Transgender People," Equality NC.org, May 10, 2021. https://equalitync.org/news/the_epidemic_of_violence_against_transgender_people/

UN Women. n.d. "The Shadow Pandemic: Violence Against Women During COVID-19." UN Women, Accessed January 2022. https://www.unwomen.org/en/news/in-focus/in-focus-gender-equality-in-covid-19-response/violence-against-women-during-covid-19

Walker, Taylor. 2020. "A Second, Silent Pandemic: Sexual Violence in the Time of COVID-19." *Harvard Medical School Primary Care Review*, May 1, 2020. http://info.primarycare.hms.harvard.edu/review/sexual-violence-and-covid

Wamsley, Laurel. 2021. "CDC Director Declares Racism a 'Serious Public Health Threat.'" *National Public Radio*, April 8, 2021. https://www.npr.org/2021/04/08/985524494/cdc-director-declares-racism-a-serious-public-health-threat

Welch, Michael. 2011. "Counterveillance: How Foucault and the Groupe d'Information sur les Prisons Reversed the Optics." *Theoretical Criminology* 15 (3): 301–313.

Young, Iris Marion. 1990. *Justice and the Politics of Difference*. Princeton: Princeton University Press.

Zigo, Tom. 2017. "Lambda Legal Applauds Rep. Allison's Resolution Calling for Better Policies to Protect Transgender Americans." *Lambda Legal*, September 28, 2017. https://www.lambdalegal.org/news/dc_20170928_lambda-legal-applauds-resolution-for-better-trans-protections

Zurn, Perry. 2019a. "Social Death." In *50 Concepts for a Critical Phenomenology*, eds. Gayle Salamon, Ann Murphy, and Gail Weiss, 309–314. Evanston: Northwestern University Press.

Zurn, Perry. 2019b. "Waste Culture and Isolation: Prisons, Toilets, and Gender Segregation." *Hypatia* 34 (4): 668–689.

10

EDUCATION AS BIOETHICS

Oppression and Pandemic Public Education

Kevin Timpe

Introduction

A central feature of the COVID-19 pandemic, especially in, roughly, the first six to eight months, was uncertainty. What was the best way to slow the spread of the virus? What would prove most effective in treating infection? How should public health be weighed against other goods? How long would it take to develop a vaccine? Naomi Zack (2021) has recently referred to these uncertainties as the 'epistemological dimension' of the pandemic (1) (see also Lindemann Nelson 2022 and Brynjarsdottir 2022). During the early months of the pandemic, this lack of good information about the virus made initial responses in the realms of medical and public policy difficult. Writing in November of 2020, Samuel Levine, Director of the Jewish Law Institute and Professor of Law at Touro University, noted that

> despite the overwhelmingly confusing and confounding aspects of the crisis, certain preliminary conclusions appear to have emerged [as early as Nov 2020], including a recognition of the disparate impact of the virus on some segments of the American populace. Specifically, it seems fair to say that vulnerable populations have been disproportionally impacted by the COVID-19 national crisis.
>
> *(Levine 2020, 81)*

As Vanessa Wills (2022) recently put it, the COVID-19 pandemic is "a complex of systemic social failures" (4). The pandemic not only *reveals* but *exacerbates* many of the underlying systemic problems that run throughout our present social structures.

In many ways, the pandemic has been a bioethical disaster. E. L. Quarantelli (1985), a sociologist known for his work on disasters, defines bioethical disasters as

> ad hoc, irregular occasions that involve a crisis; there is relative consensus that things have to be done, but the wherewithal is not enough to meet the demand. In a disaster, there is considerable variation in how the everyday capability/resource and demand/need balance gets unbalanced.
>
> *(50)*

DOI: 10.4324/9781003502623-14

Everyone was affected by the disaster, though not equally. While wealth couldn't fully insulate individuals from the effects of the pandemic, wealthy individuals and families tended to have a number of advantages when it came to the pandemic: increased ability to stockpile supplies, easier and quicker access to COVID testing, second homes to escape to, etc (see Kelly 2020). Wealthy and middle-class families with school-aged children were more likely to form 'educational pods,' two or three families arranging to share risk and responsibilities for the sake of their children's education, to offset some of the demand of having to suddenly instruct children from home (Moyer 2020). Access to reliable, in-home high-speed internet and computer technology would also prove to be valuable but uneven.

Many of the impacts of the pandemic obviously fall under the rubric of bioethics even though there isn't a unitary view of the field's domain. Some take it to be a narrow discipline, extending only so far as the various moral issues that arise within medical research and healthcare. But others think of bioethics as much broader. Jackie Leach Scully (2015), for instance, suggests we should understand bioethics "to include public health issues and areas of social care that interact with medical and life sciences." Along with the more usual topics of medical and research ethics, Scully lists issues of public health, family and social care, and social and cultural aspects of disability and embodiment among the topics that fall under the purview of bioethics. All of these intersect in terms of the bioethical implications of education, particularly during a global pandemic when there is no clear demarcation between educational environment and health risk. Navigating bioethical issues well requires access to needed educational resources.

The two-fold focus of this chapter is to think of education during the pandemic as a bioethical issue and to argue that much special education, especially during the early days of the pandemic, amounted to a form of oppression. The World Health Organization's Universal Declaration of Human Rights (1948) states that "everyone has the right to education" (Article 26). This right is supposed to be held "without distinction of any kind, such as race, colour, sex, language, religion, political or other opinion, national or social origin, property, birth or other aspects [including disability status]" (Article 22). A hallmark of US civil rights law is that education is "perhaps the most important function of state and local governments" (Brown v. Board of Education 1954). But the right to receive an education was significantly threatened by the pandemic across the world.[1] While access to education for both disabled and non-disabled populations was affected, the impact was not equal. This inequality is also found in other areas of the pandemic. A number of bioethicists have written about how "the COVID-19 pandemic … highlighted systemic disadvantages that people with disabilities face in the health care system" (Guidry-Grimes et al. 2020, 28). The ableism rooted in our healthcare systems combined with the increased risks to disabled populations amounts to a kind of "double jeopardy for marginalization" (Sabatello et al. 2020, 1523). Cognitively disabled individuals, for instance, were at increased risk of infection, in part because they were more likely housed in group settings, at even twice to three times the infection rate as seniors. Many of these individuals have pre-existing conditions that added to their risk. Individuals with intellectual and developmental disabilities were six times as likely to get ill with COVID-19 and two to three times as likely as the non-disabled population to die from it if infected (Kittay 2022, 68).[2] Many aspects of the collective response to the pandemic assumed, even if latently rather than explicitly, the devaluing of disabled lives that is at the heart of ableism.

This 'disproportionate disadvantage' can also be found in the educational impacts of the pandemic (cf. Timpe 2022c). Given the way that systemic forces came together to disadvantage disabled students *as* disabled students, I argue that one of the impacts of the pandemic was the oppression of disabled populations in public education. I focus on public, as opposed to private, education for three reasons. First, there is already significant variation within public education in the United States, and adding in private education would increase the complexity of the discussion to come. Second, though related, private schools are not legally required to admit disabled students at all. As a result, the services that they receive and the legal protections students in private school are afforded are significantly constrained compared with public education contexts. Finally, restricting focus here to public education aligns with pandemic concerns regarding public health and public goods.

In what follows, I focus on the disproportionate impact on disabled students in public education settings as a whole, though I recognize there are important classed and racialized differences, among others. A full treatment would require a range of intersectional issues to be addressed given what we know about the roles that race, class, gender, immigration status, etc…play within both education and access to healthcare. Schools that were already underfunded, such as found in economically depressed areas or on tribal reservations, found it even harder to respond to the pandemic while offering quality educational options quickly to their students. Anastasia Liasidou's (2013, 2014) scholarship, for instance, focuses on how other marginalized identities compound disabled student's experiences at school.[3] A full analysis of the harms experienced by disabled students would need to take into account intersectionality, "the ways in which various forms of oppression and subordination are reciprocally reinforcing, thereby pointing to the complexity of the issues at hand, which need to be tackled in simultaneous ways in both theoretical and practical terms" (Liasidou 2013, 301). The following analysis is intended to be illustrative, even if it cannot fully encapsulate the complexity of these interlocking features.

Special Education and the Start of the Pandemic

The simple truth of the matter is that disabled students as a group are not generally well-served by public education.[4] The first federal law extending the right to a public education to disabled students was the Education for All Handicapped Children Act (EAHCA), initially enacted in 1975. Its passage was, in part, a response to a congressional investigation that found that less than half of the country's 8 million disabled children were receiving an appropriate education and that nearly 25% weren't receiving any public education at all. The EAHCA was updated in 1990 and became the Individuals with Disabilities Education Act (IDEA), which was in turn updated in both 1997 and 2004. IDEA guarantees disabled children the right to a 'free appropriate public education' (FAPE). Furthermore, it requires that education be provided in the 'least restrictive environment' (LRE)—that is, for them to be educated with non-disabled students in the general education setting to the maximum extent appropriate.

However, given federalism, it is not the federal Department of Education that implements IDEA. Instead, each state develops its own application of IDEA. A state's special education program is then implemented through that state's local school districts. Each state also determines its own level and method of funding special education in public schools. As parents and educational analysts have reported for decades, the quality of education that disabled students receive unfortunately often depends on the zip code that the family lives in (Klein 2017). High property values can impact the quality of teachers, facilities, and the range of opportunities for students in public schools. Furthermore, wealthier parents are able to devote more time and resources to their children's education even outside of school. Sociologist Sean Reardon argues that the current economic achievement gap is about twice as large as the achievement gap due to race (Reardon 2011).

Given the federalist approach to public education, when the pandemic hit during the spring of 2020, it was up to individual districts to implement the policies and guidance issued by their state's department of education. In fact, the United States was one of only six countries that left decisions regarding school closings to be made at more local levels (Levinson 2020, 4). The others did so at the national level, increasing the consistency of the response within their national boarders. Unsurprisingly, district and state responses in the United States varied widely.

Nevertheless, many patterns emerged. The first school district to close to in-person instruction was Northshore School District, near Seattle, WA, on March 5, 2020. Within a week they stopped providing instruction altogether, citing special education services and their inability to "meet the strict guidelines outlined in federal and state regulations" (Northshore School District 2020). Under IDEA, public schools need to provide all qualifying students with a disability a 'free appropriate education' in the 'least restrictive environment.' This includes appropriate curriculum and educational opportunities and needed therapy services, but also equal opportunity to participate in nonacademic and extracurricular services such as athletics, student clubs, and recreational activities. Northshore thus became the first district to stop providing instruction to any students because of, in significant part, concerns about their inability to provide disabled students with what federal law requires districts to provide. An avalanche of similar closings, and similar justifications, soon followed. Ohio was the first to close all public schools at the state rather than district level on March 12. Their initiative cascaded across the country, with 15 other states following suit within a day. By early May, all but two states (Wyoming and Montana) closed schools for the rest of the academic year ("The Coronavirus Spring" 2020). School closures directly impacted over 50 million public school students in the United States.

How states could respond depended on the laws already in place. An extant New Jersey state law, for instance, prohibited offering any special educational services via telecommunications or other distance-learning tools, thereby ruling out IEPs via Zoom or other technology. Other states decided to wait and see how best to respond as the pandemic progressed. In their initial spring 2020 response, Delaware public school districts "balked at the idea of remote learning [during the pandemic] out of fear of being sued, especially related to meeting the needs of special education services" (Alamdari 2020). A similar response could be found in Kentucky. Many districts in multiple states didn't attempt to provide special education services during the initial weeks of the pandemic, hoping for a return to regular in-person instruction.

But we know that didn't happen. Meira Levinson, of Harvard's Edmond J. Safra Center for Ethics, writes that rather than finding ways to provide special education services in pandemic-appropriate ways, many states and districts decided to instead "level down to offer no educational services to anyone rather than violate principles of equity as policymakers understood them" (Levinson 2020, 6). If a district considered the education it offered through virtual or distance learning modalities to be official instructional time, then they would be required by federal law to "abide by all IEPs, 504s, and other instructional needs of students."[5] Many of the supplemental services schools have to provide to disabled students by the IEPs—such as speech, occupational, and physical therapies—simply could not be provided remotely, and so schools announced that they would be canceling all special-education services and meetings (such as required yearly IEP meetings) until schools reopened in person.

As state departments of education looked to the federal government for guidance, they received little counsel. The federal Department of Education did excuse all states from federally required standardized testing for all students on April 2, 2020. But beyond that it didn't provide many specifics about what responses should look like at the state and district level. With regard to special education in particular, the Department of Education put out guidance that

> if an LEA [local education agency] closes its schools to slow or stop the spread of spread of COVID-19, and does not provide any educational services to the general student population, then an LEA would not be required to provide services to students with disabilities during that same period.
>
> *(U.S. Department of Education 2020a, answer A-1)*

Many state and local educational agencies took this as indicating a way to avoid needing to comply with IDEA's requirements and so stopped providing official instructional time, in part to avoid having to provide special education services.[6] This revealed clear tensions between the federal and state governments, which then-Secretary of Education Betsy DeVos tried to counter. The Department of Education's Office of Special Education and Rehabilitative Services (2020c) advised, in mid-March, that:

> To be clear: ensuring compliance with the Individuals with Disabilities Education Act (IDEA), Section 504 of the Rehabilitation Act (Section 504), and Title II of the Americans with Disabilities Act *should not prevent any school from offering educational programs through distance instruction....* [Districts] should not opt to close or decline to provide distance instruction, at the expense of students, to address matters pertaining to services for students with disabilities.[7]
>
> *(emphasis added)*

This did not reassure schools. Within days of the above guidance from the Department of Education, the American Association of School Superintendents (2020) cautioned that

> it's one thing for ED [the US Department of Education] to understand this but another for Courts to understand this is the case. The law is still the law, and ED's suggestion that districts are responsible for "still meet[ing] their legal obligations by providing children with disabilities equally effective alternate access to the curriculum or services provided to other students" will be an insurmountable challenge for some districts.

This hesitancy makes sense, especially given that the Department of Education said that it would not provide waivers "for any of the core tenets of the IDEA or Section 504 of the Rehabilitation Act of 1973, most notably a free appropriate public education (FAPE) in the least restrictive environment (LRE)" (DeVos 2020, 11). It is hard to see the administration's response as little more than doublespeak, requiring of schools what the administration in no way equipped them to provide. As a result, as Samuel Levine (2020) has documented, "by nearly all accounts, the reality of special education during COVID-19 has largely ranged from inconsistent to virtually nonexistent" (82).

These tensions continued. The first federal guidance on reopening schools in the fall of 2020 was given on May 20, 2020. State and local educational agencies were hesitant to reopen too quickly, especially given the uncertainty regarding vaccine timeline and efficacy, treatment, and possibility of 'flattening the curve' that continued. Then-president Trump, on March 31, said that "[the pandemic] is going to go away, hopefully at the end of the month. And, if not, hopefully it will be soon after that" (Wolfe and Dale 2020). In early July of 2020, eager to get the country back to normal, Trump threatened to cut off all federal funding for schools that didn't resume face-to-face instruction in the fall. Secretary of Education DeVos would publicly disagree the next day, thereby adding to public uncertainty around education in the pandemic (2022). Changes that were initially intended to be stop-gap measures during the initial spring of the pandemic would sometimes last for as long as 18 months as the pandemic continued. Many public-school districts didn't return to the physical classroom until vaccines were available for teachers well into the 2020-2021 school year, and some wouldn't open for in-person instruction until 2021-2022 ("Schools Reopen" 2021).

Oppressive Educational Pressures During the Pandemic

Reflecting on the pandemic, DeVos has noted that "too many school districts failed to teach students even close to adequately once schools closed—worse yet, too many of them just didn't try" (DeVos 2022, 237). What these comments don't note, however, is that one reason that districts 'didn't try' is that they were caught between conflicting pressures without being given the resources need to alleviate either of them. The way they handled these pressures, then, resulted in actions that plausibly negatively impacted most students but disproportionately affected disabled students.

Education scholars Susan Baglieri and Priya Lalvani (2020) write that, even apart from the additional pressures caused by a pandemic, "disabled students experience layers of disadvantage and overlapping forms of oppression that are left unaddressed in educational policy and practice" (20). There are many contributing factors. The first is the chronic underfunding of special education. When passed, Congress promised to cover 40% of the additional costs of special education from federal funding. However, it has never been funded at that level and other than one year—2009, when additional funds were given as part of the recession stimulus—it has never been funded at even half of that level.[8] IDEA is thus an 'unfunded mandate' that requires schools and districts to provide services that end up coming out of general funds. It's no surprise, then, that even though the law does not allow services to be denied due to a lack of funding, it is often economic rather than pedagogical reasons that dictate the level of services. In addition to economics, there are other reasons for the disadvantage of disabled students. Even though the default location for disabled students to receive their public education is supposed to be the general education setting, and we should thus expect all teachers to have disabled students at some point, fewer than 40 states require teachers to take coursework in special education (Geiger 2006). Many states are not able to find enough teachers with sufficient training in special education settings, resulting in a shortage of qualified special education teachers.

Tens of thousands of complaints are filed every year alleging that public schools are failing to provide students with a free appropriate education in the least restrictive environment.[9] According to state and federal reporting, the majority of states fail to live up to the requirements of IDEA. Each year, the US Department of Education issues a determination for each state, based on State Performance Plans and Annual Performance Reports, which "evaluates the State's efforts to implement the requirements and purposes of the IDEA" (U.S. Department of Education 2022a). The Department of Education assigns states to one of four groups, depending on their determination:

- **meets** the requirements and purposes of IDEA;
- **needs assistance** in implementing the requirements of IDEA;
- **needs intervention** in implementing the requirements of IDEA; or
- **needs substantial intervention** in implementing the requirements of IDEA (U.S. Department of Education 2022a).

In the 2022 determination report of state implementation of IDEA, fewer than half of the states (21) were found to meet the requirements and purposes (U.S. Department of Education 2022a). While 28 states were found to satisfy IDEA in 2017, that number declined to 21 or 22 in each year between 2018 and 2021. So even apart from the pandemic, there's a history of major failure for state departments of education and local school districts achieving what's required by a 48-year-old law.

The situation in which disabled students find themselves regarding education in the United States amounts to a form of oppression. Marilyn Frye (1983) argues that oppression happens when a system constrains the relevant options for individuals, restricting what they can do given social forces:

> The experience of oppressed people is that the living of one's life is confined and shaped by forces and barriers which are not accidental or occasional and hence avoidable, but are systematically related to each other in such a way as to catch one between and among them and restrict or penalize motion in any direction. It is the experience of being caged in: all avenues, in every direction, are blocked or booby trapped.
>
> *(4)*

Frye illustrates oppressive systems using the metaphor of a birdcage: when examined individually, no single wire prevents the bird in a cage from flying away. It is only when one steps back and takes a macroscopic view of the wires *as a whole* that one realizes that they form "a network of systematically related barriers" (5). Oppression is, on her view, a macroscopic phenomenon:

> It is now possible to grasp one of the reasons why oppression can be hard to see and recognize: one can study the elements of an oppressive structure with great care and some good will without seeing the structure as a whole, and hence without seeing or being able to understand that one is looking at a cage and that there are people there who are caged, whose motion and mobility are restricted, whose lives are shaped and reduced.
>
> *(5)*

While all of us face limitations and frustrations, on Frye's account of oppression only those who in virtue of their membership in some group or category are in a social structure that encloses and reduce their options as a whole that are oppressed. Consider the reduction of options for disabled students. As mentioned earlier, it is legal for a private school to deny disabled students an opportunity for private education simply on the basis of their disability status. However, decades of data show that disabled students are regularly denied proper access to public education and all the services that are supposed to be included as required by law. When they are not given a free appropriate education, it is up to their parents to file complaints and push for improvement (see Laviano and Swanson 2017). The opportunities for education are reduced and shaped by how educational access is structured.

Similarly, Iris Marion Young (1988) also treats oppression as the result of interlocking social pressures and forces. Young draws on Frye's work but gives a more detailed account of what the structural nature of oppression looks like. Oppression need not be restricted to "the exercise of tyranny by a ruling group" (271). Unlike discrimination, which she takes to be an individualist concept, Young thinks that oppression is a systemic and structural phenomenon that can happen in the absence of bad intentions:

> Oppression in the structural sense is part of the basic fabric of a society, not a function of a few people's choice or politics.... Oppression is the inhibition of a group through a vast network of everyday practices, attitudes, assumptions, behaviors, and institutional rules. Oppression is structural or systemic. The systemic character of oppression implies that an oppressed group need not have a correlate oppressing group. While structural oppression in our society involves relations among groups, these relations do not generally fit the paradigm of one group's consciously and intentionally keeping another down.[10]
>
> *(271, 275)*

Young doesn't think that oppression is a single unified phenomenon with necessary and jointly sufficient conditions; there is no single attribute or set of attributes that all oppressed people have in common, no one "essential definition of oppression" (276).[11] She examines five different kinds of, or 'faces of,' oppression: exploitation, marginalization, powerlessness, cultural imperialism, and violence. While a case can be made that disabled individuals face all five faces of oppression,[12] here I want to examine the response to the pandemic in terms of how public education inhibited disabled students from receiving education to the same degree as non-disabled students did, contributing to their marginalization.

Given how special education actually plays out in districts and schools, it is reasonable to claim that many disabled students are oppressed by the American educational system.[13] But what I think is especially clear is that the pandemic placed various additional constraints and pressures on schools that resulted, even if unintentionally, in the indubitable oppression of disabled students. There are a range of ways that schools' practices, attitudes, assumptions, and behaviors in response to the pandemic inhibited disabled students. The following list is illustrative but doesn't aim to be exhaustive.

Many of the services and supports that disabled students rely on for accessing their public education were not easily transferred to online or remote delivery. Some were not able to be transferred at all. For instance, much of the modified content that some disabled students received was not delivered in a timely manner, especially as teachers struggled early to transition their general content to online delivery. Students with intellectual disabilities didn't receive modified curriculum. Accessible virtual instruction was often not available for blind, deaf, or deaf-blind students. Paraprofessional aid support that some students need in order to access their education couldn't be provided virtually, a lack which became very clear especially for parents also trying to work from home. Speech, physical, occupational, and other therapies often couldn't be delivered virtually, including for those students whose parents could help, yet didn't have the proper training. Mental health services couldn't be accessed, even as the need for them increased (see Turner 2021 and Morando-Rhim and Ekin 2021).

The disruption to schooling was itself a source of difficulty for some disabled students. Many autistics, for instance, thrive on routine and sameness. This is, in part, a way for them to filter out overwhelming amounts of sensory input:

> [I]t feels overwhelming to [some neurodivergent] kids because their brain connections take in too much of all this information. They can't integrate it and filter in what's important and filter out what's irrelevant....So, the world kind of feels like an extra loud, bright, over-whelming place. And that's one reason why kids develop such a fear of [or aversion to] new things, the neophobia, because they don't want to have to suddenly learn a brand-new environment and all these brand-new faces. And that's why sameness feels so good, because the same food or the same house that looks or tastes exactly the same way every time is comforting. All of these big changes around COVID have been especially disruptive for kids with autism'.
>
> *(Engel 2020)*

The change in routine, even if unavoidable given the public health concerns, had increased negative effects on autistic students beyond those experienced by students in general. Increased screen time, especially time that was to be spent on schoolwork while parents often worked in other rooms or at in-person jobs that hadn't been moved online, was also sometimes problem-atic. Such additional time, especially when it was unsupervised due to parents having to work, was sometimes used for other pursuits (e.g., YouTube, gaming, online gambling, pornogra-phy) rather than education. But even when it was directed at education, virtual education is simply unable to serve many disabled children in the same way that in-person instruction can because of how their disabilities impact their ability to engage through technology.[14] Bringing many of these threads together, Levine (2020) concludes that

> the inability to obtain effective treatment, the sudden and drastic interruption of any sense of routine, and ongoing and increasing sense of uncertainty, and seemingly ubiquitous reports of a lethal pandemic have all combined to produce substantially adverse mental health outcomes from many individuals with development disabilities.
>
> *(86)*

Many of the pandemic changes thus compounded mental health challenges that are already higher among disabled children when compared to their non-disabled peers, at least with respect to some kinds of disabilities.[15]

So even if the shift to virtual learning was justified given the epistemic uncertainty of trans-mission and risk at the time (as I think it was),[16] closing schools to mitigate the threat to public health and decrease the death toll had significant costs to students. These costs were not born equally by disabled and non-disabled students.

School and district decisions to end official instruction also show the oppressive structures constraining disabled students. If districts remained open, disabled students would have failed to get the education they are due by state and federal law since many special education ser-vices couldn't be delivered virtually, thereby opening themselves up to remedial legal action.

But the federal government had advised that "if a school district closes its schools and does not provide any education to the general student population, then a school would not be required to provide services to students with disabilities during that same period of time" (U.S. Department of Education 2020b, 11). By suspending official instruction in favor of merely offering optional supplemental learning resources, districts thus didn't have to provide any of the required services or pay attention to accessibility concerns. Both options would harm disabled students. When the options were made clear to them, one director of special education described the second route as "a game changer"[17] since it would free the district from being "crushed with compliance" with state and federal law.[18] In order to avoid the requirements of state and federal law regarding providing a free appropriate education to disabled students, districts across the country decided to discontinue official instruction for the spring of 2020. And many of these districts then didn't provide these optional supplemental learning resources in accessible formats since they were not required to do so by law.

A macroscopic view of how public schools approached special education during the pandemic shows that disabled students' options were reduced beyond those of non-disabled students. Even if this was not the intent and a result of understandable pressures caused by the pandemic, federal, state, and district decisions and policy choices inhibited the options of disabled students in ways that disproportionately disadvantaged them. As schools closed down for spring 2020 and even as Secretary of Education DeVos declared it to be "increasingly clear that students were being harmed by not being in school," the Department of Education, state departments of education, and local school districts did little to ensure that disabled students were given proper educational access (DeVos 2022, 339).

But this mistreatment didn't end when schools eventually returned to in-person instruction. As schools began to reopen in the fall of 2020, little was done to catch up for disabled students. One of the three reasons in IDEA for extended school year services (i.e., official instructional opportunities provided over the summer) is regression of skills related to a student's annual goals. While many disabled students experienced regression during the pandemic shut-down (Engel 2020 and Kamenetz 2020), the federal Department of Education has not ensured that state-level departments of education and local districts have done the needed reviews to determine the extent of regression and then provide extended school year services.

Taken together, the structural response of public education systems to the pandemic shows a systematically related set of decisions, policies, and incentives that constrained educational options and possibilities for disabled students beyond what students as a whole faced. As with other aspects of the pandemic, the response of the public education system both revealed and exacerbated ableist tendencies that disproportionately disadvantaged those with disabilities.

Conclusion

In addition to the individual and cultural ableist attitudes that many disabled individuals must face, the pandemic also revealed the *structural and institutional* ableism that disabled individuals endure. This was evidenced not only by discriminatory public health policies, but also by the responses of educational institutions. As Anna Gotlib (2022) writes about how different groups experienced the pandemic, "their disorientations, the traumas, differ in part because of the injustices inherent in our political and socioeconomic systems" (xviii). Contrary to some of the public calls that "we're all in this together," in a number of ways the pandemic has shown that such a sentiment is overly simplistic. "If anything, the coronavirus pandemic has revealed the differences in our society more than our similarities. Extreme pressure, applied to a society, a diamond or an individual mind, eventually exposes all the hidden cracks" (Engel 2020). The effects of these cracks are not equally felt. While even under the best of conditions disabled students often face institutional ableism,[19] school's responses sometimes introduce new levels of institutional ableism and oppression.

Elizabeth Anderson (2012) reminds us that "structural injustices call for structural remedies" (171). We need a social justice approach to education policy even apart from public health crises; but the pandemic has highlighted the need for such an approach. It has revealed how we actually do, socially, value (or devalue) lives. Public schools' responses to the pandemic show that they were willing to magnify existing inequalities rather than seek to provide the best educational opportunities for all students. While there is a "mediating role that schools [could] play in alleviating social inequalities and minimizing the achievement gap between privileged and disadvantaged groups of students," what actually happened during the COVID-19 pandemic in the United States was a compounding of previous inequalities that in some cases amounted to oppression (Liasidou 2013, 306). While many bioethicists have noted how this happened with regard to health-care resources and access, disabled people's health and well-being were also harmed by the country's educational response to COVID-19.

Given the interconnections between education and various dimensions of social care, we should think more fully about education as a locus of bioethics, even apart from the pandemic. What could be done to prevent similar results in the future? A complete answer to this question would require another essay, but a number of key pieces stand out. First, IDEA should be fully funded so that state departments of education and local school districts no longer have such a large financial incentive to scrimp on special education services, even apart from a pandemic. Second, districts would have benefitted from clearer federal guidance. There is also a significant need for greater accountability for school districts. This includes extended school year evaluation, regression prevention, and recoupment. Even though districts chose to provide supplemental learning resources as a way of avoiding the demands of IDEA that would have been in place had they been providing official instruction, to minimize the educational harm to specifically disabled students districts should also explore the need for compensatory educational services for missed instructional time and their failure to provide a free appropriate education during the pandemic.[20] All of these steps could have, if taken by districts in response to the pandemic, minimized the long-term educational impact on disabled students. But especially given the financial point earlier coupled with the limited options for holding public districts accountable for failing to live up to the requirements of IDEA even apart from a global pandemic, districts have, and short of considerable change in educational policy will continue to have, perverse incentives to oppress disabled students will likely continue.[21]

Notes

1   See the discussions, for instance, of England and India in Weale 2020 and Pandey and Srivastava 2020, respectively. Despite the impact of the pandemic on education being a global phenomenon, the remainder of the article focuses simply on the United States.

2   See Levine 2020 and Shapiro 2020. Other groups marginalized by our culture also had increased risk, including racial minorities and native and indigenous populations; see, for instance, Abbasi 2020 and Yancey 2020.

3 See also Goodley and Runswick-Cole 2010 for a discussion of how disability compounds with other forms of exclusion into a web of social disadvantage.

4 Given that they are exempt from the Individuals with Disabilities Education Act, private schools do not have to admit disabled students much less provide them accommodations and supports in the same way that federal law requires for public schools. In fact, private schools can deny disabled students admission simply on the basis of a student having a disability. Parents of disabled students who do attend private schools often have to take whatever supports and accommodations the school is willing to provide; pushing too hard for further services, which IDEA and state procedural safeguards provide a route for in public school, can result in private schools simply removing the offer of admission, forcing the student to find another school to attend. The situation is thus often even more problematic for disabled students in such educational settings.

5 Richfield Public Schools Distance Learning Comprehensive Guide for Staff; March 18, 2020. Obtained via Freedom of Information Act request. See also Levine 2020, 11.

6 I discuss this in considerable detail using Grand Rapids Public Schools as an example in Timpe 2022c.

7 Looking back on this early response, DeVos has more recently claimed that "Congress didn't want to take the blame for shortchanging students with disabilities. So, they punted to me. They gave me thirty days to decide if there would be a waiver on meeting the requirements of the IDEA" (DeVos 2022, 250). There wouldn't be such a waiver. But DeVos's Department of Education also didn't provide additional guidance on how to satisfy those requirements in the middle of a pandemic, instead punting instead to state and local educational agencies.

8 The 2021 funding level, for instance, was only 17% of the additional cost to serve disabled students.

9 During the 2018-2019 school year, there were 5,575 written signed complaints; 21,338 due process complaints; and 11,671 mediation requests filed (43rd Annual Report to Congress on the Implementation of IDEA 2021, xxxi). As indicated in the report, "the year in the title reflects the U.S. Department of Educations's target year for submitting the report to Congress. The most current data in this report were collected from July 2018 through December 2019" (xv, footnote 1). It will take a few years for the data from the pandemic to be reflected in this annual report.

10 More specifically, as the latter part of this quotation indicates, Young thinks people are oppressed in terms of their group affinity, where one just *finds* oneself to be a member of a group, and not just membership in a voluntary association.

11 Elsewhere, I have argued that something similar is true of the concept of disability; see Timpe 2022b.

12 For a discussion of cultural imperialism, with a specific focus on communicative norms, see Reynolds and Timpe 2024 and Timpe 2022a. For discussions of violence against disabled people, see Shapiro 1994 and McGuire 2016.

13 While Young explicitly describes both marginalization and exploitation in terms of work, the spirit of her treatment also applies to educational access and opportunity. I thank Barrett Emerick for bringing this point to my attention.

14 While some students, including some disabled students, benefitted from online instruction and virtual learning, that doesn't mean that disabled students as a group were not oppressed. See also Levine 2020, 84 note 8.

15 See, for instance Breslau 1985. Eric Emerson's research, for instance, has found that particularly intellectual disability correlates with "significantly increased risk of certain forms of psychiatric disorder" (Emerson 2003, 51) with an odds ratio of 4.8 for PTSD, 2.9 for panic disorder, 2.6 for generalized anxiety, and 1.7 for depression (54).

16 Here, as elsewhere, however there is a concern that the public health response to the pandemic encouraged thinking about public health primarily through a medical lens, often downplaying some of the social factors that are equally important for public health. While attempting to address public health, decisions were made that further individualized education and reduced the social care educational institutions at their best can provide.

17 Email from Laura LaMore to SE Admin—LOCAL Supervisors, May 23, 2020, 11:50 am. Obtained via Freedom of Information Act request.

18 Email from Laura LaMore to Richard Lemons, May 20, 2020, 4:52 pm. Obtained via Freedom of Information Act request.

19 See Baglieri and Lalvani 2020, particularly chapter 1 and Dolmage 2017.

20 For initial moves in this direction, see *Education Law Center* 2022 and *U.S. Department of Education* 2022b.

21 Thanks to Kate Strater, Barrett Emerick, Alison Reiheld, Anna Gotlib, and Alida Liberman for conversations and interactions that shaped this chapter for the better. Their input, however, doesn't indicate agreement with what I here write. And I am especially grateful for the input and guidance of the editors of this volume, Mercer Gary and Joel Michael Reynolds, for both significant input and the opportunity to be a part of this volume.

Works Cited

Abbasi, Jennifer. 2020. "Taking a Closer Look at COVID-19, Health Inequities, and Racism." *JAMA Network*, June 29, 2020. https://jamanetwork.com/journals/jama/fullarticle/2767948

Alamdari, Natalia. 2020. "Delaware Public Schools are Beginning Remote Learning. But Should They Fear Future Lawsuits?" *Delaware Online*, April 1, 2020. https://www.delawareonline.com/story/news/2020/04/01/coronavirus-should-delaware-schools-fear-lawsuits-remote-learning-begins/5094015002/

Anderson, Elizabeth. 2012. "Epistemic Justice as a Virtue of Social Institutions." *Social Epistemology* 26 (2):163–173.

Baglieri, Susan, and Priya Lalvani. 2020. *Undoing Ableism*. New York: Routledge.

Breslau, Naomi. 1985. "Psychiatric Disorder in Children with Physical Disabilities." *Journal of the American Academy of Child Psychiatry* 24 (1): 87–94.

Brynjarsdottir, Eyja M. 2022. "The COVID-19 Guidebook for Living in an Alternate Universe." In *Responses to a Pandemic: Philosophical and Political Reflections*, edited by Anna Gotlib, 189–200. Lanham, MD: Rowman & Littlefield.

DeVos, Betsy. 2020. "Recommended Waiver Authority Under Section 3511(d)(4) of Division A of the Coronavirus Aid, Relief, and Economic Security Act ('CARES Act')." *U.S. Department of Education*. https://www2.ed.dov/documents/coronavirus/cares-waiver-report.pdf

DeVos, Betsy. 2022. *Hostages No More: The Fight for Educational Freedom and the Future of the American Child*. Nashville, TN: Center Street.

Dolmage, Jay Timothy. 2017. *Academic Ableism: Disability and Higher Education*. Ann Arbor, MI: University of Michigan Press.

"ED Issues Guidance on FAPE During COVID-19." 2020. *The School Superintendents Association*. http://web.archive.org/web/20210917042059/https://www.aasa.org/policy-blogs.aspx?id=44560&blogid=84002

Education Law Center. 2022. "New Law Protects Pandemic-Related Compensatory Education for NJ Students with Disabilities." March 9, 2022. https://edlawcenter.org/news/archives/special-education/new-law-protects-pandemic-related-compensatory-education-for-nj-students-with-disabilities.html

Emerson, Eric. 2003. "Prevalence of Psychiatric Disorders in Children and Adolescents with and Without Intellectual Disability." *Journal of Intellectual Disability Research* 47 (1): 51–58.

Engel, Richard 2020. "Kids with Special Needs are Not OK Right Now. Neither are Parents." *Today*, August 10, 2020. https://www.yahoo.com/now/richard-engel-kids-special-needs-230000057.html

Frye, Marilyn. 1983. "Oppression." In *Politics of Reality: Essays in Feminist Theory*, 1–16. New York: Crossing Press.

Geiger, Willieam L. 2006. *A Compilation of Research on States' Licensure Models for Special Education Teachers and Special Education Requirements for Licensing General Education Teachers*. Washington, DC: Educational Resources Information Center Clearinghouse.

Goodley, Dan, and Katherine Runswick-Cole. 2010. "Len Barton, Inclusion and Critical Disability Studies: Theorising Disabled Childhoods." *International Studies in Sociology of Education* 20 (4): 273–290.

Gotlib, Anna. 2022. "*In Medias Res*: Philosophers as Witnesses to Disaster." In *Responses to a Pandemic: Philosophical and Political Reflections*, edited by Anna Gotlib, xiii–xxiv. Lanham, MD: Rowman & Littlefield.

Guidry-Grimes, Laura, Katie Savin, Joseph A. Stramondo, Joel Michael Reynolds, Marina Tsaplina, Teresa Blankmeyer Burke, Angela Ballantyne, Eva Feder Kittay, Devan Stahl, Jackie Leach Scully, Rosemaria Garland-Thomson, Anita Tarzian, Doraon Dorfman, and Joseph J. Fins. 2020. "Disability Rights as a Necessary Framework for Crisis Standards of Care and the Future of Healthcare." *The Hastings Center Report* 50 (3): 28–32. https://onlinelibrary.wiley.com/doi/abs/10.1002/hast.1128

Kamenetz, Anya. 2020. "Families of Children with Special Needs are Suing in Several States. Here's Why." *National Public Radio*, July 23, 2020. https://www.npr.org/2020/07/23/893450709/families-of-children-with-special-needs-are-suing-in-several-states-heres-why

Kelly, Jack. 2020. "The Rich are Riding Out the Coronavirus Pandemic Very Differently than the Rest of Us." *Forbes*, April 1, 2020. https://www.forbes.com/sites/jackkelly/2020/04/01/the-rich-are-riding-out-the-coronavirus-pandemic-very-differently-than-the-rest-of-us/

Kittay, Eva Feder. 2022. "The Nightmare of Triage and Discrimination: Whose Benefit Is to Be Maximized?" In *Responses to a Pandemic: Philosophical and Political Reflections*, edited by Anna Gotlib, 67–75. Lanham, MD: Rowman & Littlefield.

Klein, Rebecca. 2017. "For Students with Disabilities, Quality of Education can Depend on Zip Code." *The Hechinger Report*, December 19, 2017. https://hechingerreport.org/students-disabilities-quality-education-can-depend-zip-code/

Laviano, Jennifer and Julie Swanson. 2017. *Your Special Education Rights: What Your School District Isn't Telling You.* New York: Skyhorse Publishing.

Levine, Samuel J. 2020. "COVID-19 and Individuals with Developmental Disabilities: Tragic Realities and Cautious Hope." *Arizona State Law Journal* 2: 80–89.

Levinson, Meira. 2020. "Educational Ethics During a Pandemic." *Edmond J. Safra Center for Ethics at Harvard University*. https://ethics.harvard.edu/files/center-for-ethics/files/17educationalethics2.pdf

Liasidou, Anastasia. 2013. "Intersectional Understandings of Disability and Implications for a Social Justice Reform Agenda in Education Policy and Practice." *Disability & Society* 28 (3): 299–312.

Liasidou, Anastasia. 2014. "Critical Disability Studies and Socially Just Change in Higher Education." *British Journal of Special Education* 41 (2):120–135.

Lindemann Nelson, Jamie. 2022. "We Survived COVID-19! (Possibly)." In *Responses to a Pandemic: Philosophical and Political Reflections*, edited by Anna Gotlib, 103–114. Lanham, MD: Rowman & Littlefield.

McGuire, Anne. 2016. *War on Autism: On the Cultural Logic of Normative Violence.* Ann Arbor, MI: University of Michigan Press.

Morando-Rhim, Lauren and Sumeyra Ekin. 2021. "How Has the Pandemic Affected Students with Disabilities? A Review of the Evidence to Date." *The Center on Reinventing Public Education*. https://crpe.org/wp-content/uploads/final_swd_report_2021.pdf

Moyer, Melinda Wenner. 2020. "Pods, Microschools and Tutors: Can Parents Solve the Education Crisis on Their Own?" *The New York Times*, July 22, 2020. https://www.nytimes.com/2020/07/22/parenting/school-pods-coronavirus.html

Northshore School District. March 12, 2020. "Letter to Families: Gov. Inslee's Announcement." https://www.nsd.org/blog/~board/superintendent-blog/post/letter-to-families-gov-inslees-announcement

Pandey, Pooja and Sumyesh Srivastava. 2020. "Excluding the Excluded: India's Response to the Education of Children with Disabilities During COVID-19." *The Times of India*, April 26, 2020. https://timesofindia.indiatimes.com/blogs/voices/excluding-the-excluded-indias-response-to-the-education-of-children-with-disabilities-during-covid-19/

Quarantelli, E. L. 1985. "What Is Disaster? The Need for Clarification in Definition and Conceptualization in Research." *Disaster Research Center Report* 177: 41–73.

Reardon, Sean F. 2011. "The Widening Academic Achievement Gap Between the Rich and the Poor: New Evidence and Possible Explanations." In *Whither Opportunity? Rising Inequality, Schools, and Children's Life Chances*, edited by Greg J. Duncan and Richard J. Murnane, 91–116. New York: Russell Sage Foundation.

Reynolds, Joel Michael, and Kevin Timpe. 2024. "Disability and Knowing: On Social Epistemology's Ableism Problem." In *The Oxford Handbook of Social Epistemology*, edited by Jennifer Lackey and Aidan McGlynn. Oxford: Oxford University Press.

Sabatello, May, Teresa Blankmeyer Burke, Katherine E. McDonald, and Paul S. Appelbaum. 2020. "Disability, Ethics, and Health Care in the COVID-19 Pandemic." *Public Health Ethics* 110 (10): 1523–1527.

"Schools Reopen: Stories from Across Pandemic America." 2021. *The New York Times*, September 17, 2021. https://www.nytimes.com/2021/09/17/education/learning/schools-reopening-united-states.html

Scully, Jackie Leach. 2015. "Feminist Bioethics." In *Stanford Encyclopedia of Philosophy*, edited by Edward N. Zalta. https://plato.stanford.edu/entries/feminist-bioethics/

Shapiro, Joseph P. 1994. *No Pity*. New York: Three Rivers Press.

Shapiro, Joseph. 2020. "COVID-19 Infections and Deaths are Higher Among Those with Intellectual Disabilities." *National Public Radio*, June 9, 2020. https://www.npr.org/2020/06/09/872401607/covid-19-infections-and-deaths-are-higher-among-those-with-intellectual-disabili

"The Coronavirus Spring: The Historic Closing of U.S. Schools (a Timeline)." 2020. *Education Week*. https://www.edweek.org/leadership/the-coronavirus-spring-the-historic-closing-of-u-s-schools-a-timeline/2020/07

Timpe, Kevin. 2022a. "Cognitive Disabilities, Forms of Exclusion, and the Ethics of Social Interactions." *The Journal of Philosophy of Disability* 2: https://www.pdcnet.org/jpd/content/jpd_2022_0999_6_7_14

Timpe, Kevin. 2022b. "Denying a Unified Concept of Disability." *The Journal of Medicine and Philosophy* 47 (5): 583–596.

Timpe, Kevin. 2022c. "Disability and Disproportionate Disadvantage." In *Responses to a Pandemic: Philosophical and Political Reflections*, edited by Anna Gotlib, 77–99. Lanham, MD: Rowman & Littlefield.

Turner, Cory. 2021. "After Months of Special Education Turmoil, Families Say Schools Owe Them." *National Public Radio*, June 16, 2021. https://www.npr.org/2021/06/16/994587239/after-months-of-special-education-turmoil-families-say-schools-owe-them

U.S. Department of Education. 2020a. "Questions and Answers on Providing Services to Children with Disabilities During the Coronavirus Disease 2019 Outbreak (March 2020)." https://sites.ed.gov/idea/idea-files/q-and-a-providing-services-to-children-with-disabilities-during-the-coronavirus-disease-2019-outbreak/

U.S. Department of Education. 2020b. "Recommended Waiver Authority Under Section 3511(d)(4) of Division A of the Coronavirus Aid, Relieve, and Economic Security Act ('CARES Act')." https://www2.ed.gov/documents/coronavirus/cares-waiver-report.pdf

U.S. Department of Education. 2020c. "Supplemental Fact Sheet: Addressing the Risk of COVID-19 in Preschool, Elementary and Secondary Schools While Serving Children with Disabilities." https://www2.ed.gov/about/offices/list/ocr/frontpage/faq/rr/policyguidance/Supple%20Fact%20Sheet%203.21.20%20FINAL.pdf

U.S. Department of Education. 2022a. "2022 Determination Letters on State Implementation of IDEA." https://sites.ed.gov/idea/idea-files/2022-determination-letters-on-state-implementation-of-idea/

U.S. Department of Education. 2022b. "Office for Civil Rights Reaches Resolution Agreement with Nation's Second Largest School District, Los Angeles Unified, to Meet Needs of Students with Disabilities during COVID-19 Pandemic." https://www.ed.gov/news/press-releases/office-civil-rights-reaches-resolution-agreement-nations-second-largest-school-district-los-angeles-unified-meet-needs-students-disabilities-during-covid-19-pandemic

United Nations. 1948. "Declaration on the Rights of Disabled Persons." *United Nations*. https://www.un.org/en/about-us/universal-declaration-of-human-rights

Weale, Sally. 2020. "English Schools 'Using Coronavirus as Excuse' Not to Teach Special Education Pupils." *The Guardian*, July 1, 2020. https://www.theguardian.com/education/2020/jul/01/english-schools-using-coronavirus-as-excuse-not-to-teach-special-needs-pupils

Wills, Vanessa. 2022. "The New Normals. Solidarity, Recognition, and Vulnerable Selves in the COVID-19 Pandemic." In *Responses to a Pandemic: Philosophical and Political Reflections*, edited by Anna Gotlib, 3–17. Lanham, MD: Rowman & Littlefield.

Wolfe, Daniel and Daniel Dale. 2020. "'It's Going to Disappear': A Timeline of Trump's Claims that COVID-19 will Vanish." *CNN*, October 31, 2020. https://edition.cnn.com/interactive/2020/10/politics/covid-disappearing-trump-comment-tracker/

Yancey, Clyde W. 2020. "COVID-19 and African Americans." *Journal of the American Medical Association* 323 (19): 1891–1892.

Young, Iris Marion. 1988. "Five Faces of Oppression." *The Philosophical Forum* 19 (4): 270–290.

Zack, Naomi. 2021. *The American Tragedy of COVID-19*. Lanham, MD: Rowman & Littlefield.

11

BUILDING INSTITUTIONAL TRUSTWORTHINESS IN EMERGENCY CONDITIONS

Lessons from Disability Scholarship and Activism

Corinne Lajoie

We hear time and time again that trust in institutions is declining at alarming rates. In recent years, the COVID-19 pandemic has revealed concerning levels of distrust in medical and public health institutions. Experts suggest that restoring the public's trust in these institutions is key to ensuring successful healthcare delivery and reducing widely documented health inequities across populations. Amidst this discourse, however, an important point is too often lost. Quite simply, trust is ineffective without trustworthiness. At a practical level, placing trust in untrustworthy persons or institutions is imprudent. For members of socially marginalized groups, conditions of oppression and structural injustice raise the stakes of trust. Distrust is only rational in the face of institutional failures to reliably serve and protect members of these groups. As Onora O'Neill (2013) has famously argued, the popular claim that we need *more trust*—whether between persons, or between persons and institutions—is misleading. Instead of generalized trust, we need institutions we can reliably trust.

Building on this insight, this chapter shifts the focus from discussions of public trust to an examination of the role of *institutional trustworthiness* in addressing public health concerns and crises. I argue that medical and public health institutions have a responsibility to cultivate and demonstrate trustworthiness toward the populations they serve, especially toward oppressed and marginalized people. This requires taking concrete steps to identify, recognize, and remedy the forms of injustice entrenched in healthcare distribution and delivery and in the design of public health policies. Understanding what it means—and, centrally, what it *takes*—to be trustworthy shifts our attention away from individual attitudes of trust and distrust and toward the ethical responsibilities of institutions whose role it is to be stewards of the public good both in times of crisis and beyond them.

Mechanisms of institutional trustworthiness can be understood by examining the place of trust and trustworthiness in ethical life. The first section of this chapter briefly introduces the philosophical literature on these topics, showing how trustworthiness is connected to human need, dependency, and vulnerability. Just as they can show themselves to be trustworthy, persons and institutions can betray our trust and act in untrustworthy ways. Failures and deficiencies of trustworthiness have particularly devastating effects on the lives of marginalized and oppressed people who are already socially disenfranchised. The second section of this

DOI: 10.4324/9781003502623-15

paper considers how ableist medical triage policies adopted during COVID-19 function as examples of institutional *un*-trustworthiness. I argue that medical and public health institutions failed to protect the interests of the people who depended on them by responding to the crisis in ways that discriminated against disabled people. I end by offering four recommendations for building institutional trustworthiness in times of crisis and beyond them. These recommendations include (1) developing a robust, historically informed understanding of why oppressed and marginalized people might mistrust medical and public health institutions; (2) adopting an intersectional lens of analysis regarding the impacts of public health crises; (3) increasing clarity about the implicit norms and values driving public health policy and practice, and, finally, (4) recognizing and centering the knowledge and skills of disabled people. Throughout, my view is that oppressive systems can and do adversely affect relations of trust. The task of building institutional trustworthiness is inherently tied to the project of social transformation.

The Ethics of Trust and Trustworthiness

The philosophical literature on trust makes an important distinction between trust and reliance. Although scholars disagree about the reasons why this is the case, many agree that trust is irreducible to mere reliance (Baier 1986; Jones 2004; Potter 2002). I may rely on my car to get started in the morning, for example, but I do not typically feel a sense of betrayal if it does not. I will instead likely feel irritated or displeased. Similarly, I might implicitly rely on a friend to bring snacks on a long hike because they have the best planning skills in my entire friend group, but there is no moral expectation at stake in this scenario and I will not be 'let down,' so to speak, if my friend does not pack snacks that day. In contrast with mere reliance, trust has a salient normative force because it engages our vulnerability to others in a distinctive way.[1] The vulnerability inherent to trust is painfully revealed when a person (or, as we will later see, an institution) fails to provide or protect something we deeply value. As Annette Baier writes, "we come to realize what trust involves retrospectively and posthumously, once our vulnerability is brought home to us by actual wounds" (Baier 1986, 235). If my child suffers serious harm under the supervision of a caretaker, I will likely feel something much stronger than disappointment and more akin to betrayal. I did not merely assume that the caretaker was reliable. I trusted that they could keep my child safe and care for them in an attentive and responsive manner. In trusting others, we make ourselves vulnerable to them, and thus trust always presents a level of risk.

If trust is so dangerous, why trust at all? Trust is a ubiquitous and necessary part of life. We trust bankers not to steal all our money, bus drivers to navigate the streets safely, medical professionals to be transparent about the risks of a procedure, and friends to keep our most embarrassing secrets. As Johnny Brennan puts it, "it is impossible to withdraw trust entirely [given that we] cannot take care of all our goods (material and otherwise) at every moment" (2024, 245). We trust people all the time, in myriad ways, many of which are inapparent to us. Indeed, trust is not always (and perhaps even not often) a deliberate, self-conscious, and calculated decision. Many instances of trust are unconscious and only become apparent to us when our trust is violated. Although trusting others involves certain risks, trust also yields several benefits. It allows us to accomplish basic tasks, develop meaningful relationships, acquire knowledge, and cooperate successfully with others. Most fundamentally, trust is central to our lives as finite, social, and embodied persons who depend on others to meet a variety of needs (e.g., for shelter, sustenance, protection, education, social participation etc.). Feminist ethicists have long argued that need, vulnerability, and dependency are foundational dimensions of human existence (Butler 2004; Miller 2011; Gilson 2013; Rogers, Mackenzie, and Dodds 2012; Kittay 1999). Trust is the missing link in this picture. It can compound and alleviate each of these elements. We depend on others to meet our needs and are vulnerable to the actions (and, crucially, the *inaction*) of those we trust. Trustees can respond to need and dependency in ways that promote our agency, safety, and flourishing. On the other hand, they can neglect, abuse, or exploit the dependencies we have on them, exacerbate our vulnerability, and ignore our needs. In other words, they can prove themselves to be trustworthy or untrustworthy.

Just as there are many philosophical accounts of trust, accounts of trustworthiness differ from each other. To be trustworthy means different things depending on how one conceives trust. And, if one believes that there are many kinds of trust, then it follows that there are different senses in which a trustee can be trustworthy. My goal in this chapter is not to offer a survey of existing views regarding the nature of trustworthiness. Rather, I wish to emphasize that trustworthiness is inextricably tied to the risks involved in trust. Trust is valuable when it is warranted, but hazardous when it isn't. While in some cases it may be reasonable to trust someone with only minimal evidence of their trustworthiness (e.g., the fact that the bus driver is licensed to drive a bus is likely enough for me to assume that they can be trusted to drive it), in other instances we might want more extensive assurances of a person's trustworthiness before trusting them (e.g., if I am looking for a medical professional to treat a medically contested condition, I might ask to speak with them over the phone before booking an appointment to assess their character, consult online reviews by previous patients, and ask a friend to accompany me to my first appointment to gather their perspective). Especially when we count on them to protect the things we value most and to meet our most basic needs, we hope that the actors we trust will be trustworthy.

Placing our trust in untrustworthy actors can have devastating consequences ranging from feelings of betrayal and abandonment to loss of social networks, financial insecurity, ill health, physical injury, or even loss of life. Failures of trustworthiness are especially costly for trusters who are already made vulnerable by their relative powerlessness at a structural level. Imagine, for instance, a young female student who is abused by an older male professor who she trusted to be her mentor. Following the abuse, this student may feel that she cannot report her professor because he holds power over her and because he is more likely to be believed because of his gender and social status. In addition to experiencing physical and psychological harm, this student may find it difficult to trust professors in the future, especially if they are men, and eventually limit her participation in academic activities. In the end, she might forego the pursuit of her professional aspirations. As much as it may be valuable and even necessary, the precautionary distrust she harbors toward men in positions of authority following this incident can impede her well-being on multiple levels for many years to come.[2] Failures of trustworthiness can have damaging ripple effects that extend far beyond the scope of isolated incidents.

As this example shows, considerations of power and privilege shape the conditions of trust. As such, they should not be divorced from the study of trustworthiness. Doing so only benefits groups and individuals who are accustomed to being easily trusted and who believe they are exempt from the requirement to provide assurances of their trustworthiness. In her work on trustworthiness, Nancy Nyquist Potter (2002) suggests that "[the] self-examining question 'Why don't some people trust me?' is hardly ever asked — at least, it's seldom asked by those in positions of power with regard to the less powerful" (xi) Instead, privileged people tend to assume their own trustworthiness. Potter challenges this view and argues that in societies shaped by conditions of oppression, "persons with more privilege or power have proportionately more work to do to give assurances which provide a trustworthy character" (17). They "bear more of the responsibility to establish trustworthiness" because the possibility that they might abuse their power over the relatively powerless renders them initially less trustworthy (18). In sum, rather than conjuring *de facto* trustworthiness, social power and privilege call forth ethical responsibilities for demonstrating one's trustworthiness.

Most of the examples I have considered thus far involve trust between persons. Yet just as we place our trust in individuals, we also trust (and distrust) institutions. A minimal level of trust in institutions is important to ensure the functioning of societies. We entrust institutions with vital responsibilities, from the education of children to the promotion of scientific research, the preservation of cultural artifacts, or the protection of our democracies. Because we depend on institutions to meet some of our most basic needs, our relationships with them are sites of intense vulnerability. This is the case, for example, with medical and public health institutions. These institutions play a critical role in ensuring healthcare delivery and addressing emerging health crises. They are expected to equitably promote the health and welfare of the entire population, and especially that of groups and individuals who are most vulnerable to death, illness, or injury. Given the considerable power they hold over our lives, we hope that medical and public health institutions will protect the interests of the people they are responsible to serve. Failures of trustworthiness have particularly devastating effects on the lives of marginalized and oppressed people who are already socially disenfranchised. As the next section will show, such failures and their devastating effects on the lives of disabled people were on sharp display during the COVID-19 pandemic.

Institutional Failures of Trustworthiness During COVID-19

The themes of need, vulnerability, and dependency were multiply highlighted by the COVID-19 pandemic. In countries with developed healthcare and public health systems, individuals are dependent on these institutions for access to information, care, and services. Medical institutions have monopolies on the provision of certain kinds of care and treatment. In recent years, the proliferation of healthcare monopolies has drastically driven up medical costs for patients while often reducing quality of care (Pearl 2023; Rosalsky 2021). Patients find themselves dependent on healthcare systems that exacerbate social and financial inequalities. A public health crisis amplifies the public's dependency on medical and public health systems. At the height of the COVID-19 pandemic, many people turned to official websites like the CDC's for up-to-date information about cases numbers or recommended sanitation measures, while other people received life-saving medical attention in hospitals across the country. Disabled people experienced additional forms of vulnerability and dependency during the pandemic due to institutional failures and pervasive ableism in healthcare. For instance, disabled people and older adults living in congregate settings experienced dramatically high rates of mortality and infection. Rather than calling attention to the egregious living conditions in understaffed and underresourced facilities, however, the deaths of disabled people and older adults were "naturalized, depoliticized, and rationalized" as the inevitable consequences of their purportedly inherent vulnerability (Tremain, 2020).

In addition to being disproportionately exposed to the risk of infection due to situational factors, disabled people were met institutionally with discriminatory triage policies that exponentially amplified their vulnerability to harm. In the United States, complaints filed with the Department of Health and Human Service's Office of Civil Rights by organizations across several states (notably, Alabama, Washington, Kansas, Tennessee, Pennsylvania, Utah, New York, Oklahoma, North Carolina, and Oregon) argued that protocols for care rationing that systematically deprioritized disabled patients violated key sections of the Affordable Care Act (ACA), the Americans with Disabilities Act (ADA) and the Rehabilitation Act. In Alabama, for example, the Emergency Operations plan ordered hospitals to withhold mechanical ventilator support for patients with severe intellectual disabilities as a last resort. Meanwhile, in Tennessee, critical care guidelines denied treatment to patients with spinal muscular atrophy requiring assistance with daily tasks (Stramondo 2020; Ne'eman 2020). In Canada, the draft COVID-19 Triage Protocol circulated to Ontario hospitals in January 2021 also emphasized a patient's ability to perform daily tasks without assistance as a selection criterion for care allocation (PressProgress 2021). Triage protocols in Quebec initially included specific disabilities such as cognitive impairments and Parkinson's disease as grounds for deprioritization (Zhu et al. 2022).

The discrimination expressed by several triage policies was forcefully criticized from all corners of the disability community. Successful lawsuits were filed against states whose triage protocols discriminated against disabled people. In response, several states revised or redrafted their protocols for critical care allocation in response to critiques. Moreover, disabled writers and activists, disability groups, and disability bioethicists brought discussions of widespread rights violations and medical ableism to the forefront of public and scholarly discussions of critical care allocation (Mello, Persad, and White 2020; Reynolds, Guidry-Grimes, and Savin 2021; Solomon, Wynia, and Gostin 2020). The swift and organized response of the disability community and its allies called attention to the egregious discrimination faced daily by disabled people in the medical system and in society more broadly. Disabled activist and author Alice Wong (2020) writes of her experience as a disabled Asian American person using a ventilator during the pandemic: "Were I to contract coronavirus, I imagine a doctor might read my chart, look at me, and think I'm a waste of their efforts and precious resources." Wong's concerns resonate with the criticisms leveled above at emergency triage protocols. Her observation that frameworks for rationing care "put people like [her] at the bottom of the list" is personal and political (2020). It ties together her fear of not surviving the pandemic due to discriminatory treatment with a political awareness of the accepted social disposability of disabled people. As Wong puts it, disabled people were treated as "acceptable collateral damage" in an all-too-familiar utilitarian calculus that prioritized the lives of non-disabled people (2020).

Wong's fears of being treated as "collateral damage" are far from being unfounded. In early January 2022, the director of the Center for Disease Control and Prevention, Dr. Rachelle Walensky, delivered remarks on national television about what she termed the "encouraging news" that three-fourths of COVID-19 fatalities from the Omicron variant occurred among people who were "unwell to begin with." A few short weeks after delivering these remarks on *Good Morning America*, Dr. Walensky referred to masks as the "scarlet letter" of the pandemic on a podcast, claiming that they are both "inconvenient" and "annoying," at the same time as COVID-19 cases continued soaring across the United States. Dr. Walensky's various public blunders offer a window into the many failures in public health policy and messaging that characterized this crisis. They also reflect the conclusions advanced by the triage proto-cols discussed above. At every turn during the unfolding of the pandemic, disabled people's deaths were tacitly accepted as the price to pay to keep the wheels of able-bodied society turn-ing. Decisions about how to respond to a crisis like the one at hand are ultimately decisions about the kind of world we want to live in and the people who belong in it. The general mes-sage sent by Walensky's remarks, discriminatory hospital triage protocols, and institutional indifference to the systemic forms of harm experienced by disabled people in medical systems is that a post-pandemic world with less disabled people in it is an acceptable, and even perhaps desirable, world.

The discriminatory triage policies put forth by state and medical institutions are not only alarming because they discriminate against a legally protected class. I argue they should also worry us because they illustrate the *un*-trustworthiness of medical and public health institu-tions during COVID-19 for disabled people. In saying this, I am not merely saying that these institutions failed to demonstrate their trustworthiness. In other words, the issue at stake is not simply that we lack sufficient evidence to positively establish their trustworthiness. The issue, rather, is that these institutions showed that they are not deserving of disabled people's trust. They acted in an untrustworthy manner. Karen Jones (2012) describes trustworthiness as a particular type of response to the fact of human dependency. She explains that trustwor-thiness is "a distinctive way in which human beings can actively and positively engage with the fact of another's dependency, through their ability to recognize it" (66). On this view, being trustworthy involves both *recognizing* human dependency and *responding* to it positively by harnessing one's power to intervene in the life of another person, group, or entity. Being trust-worthy involves being responsive to the ways in which one is being counted on by dependent others in a domain in which the trustee is competent. Jones' remarks concern the case of interpersonal dependency, but they can also shed light on the relations of dependency we have with institutions. In this case, medical and public health institutions failed to carry through with their most fundamental professional and ethical obligations toward the people who depended on them during a global health emergency. Instead of *recognizing* and *responding* to this dependency by acting in ways that showed they could be counted on, medical and public health institutions prioritized the lives of nondisabled people at the expense of some of the most vulnerable sectors of the population.

For many disabled people, the institutional response to the pandemic was morally outra-geous, but not altogether surprising. The institutional response to the COVID-19 pandemic is the latest in a series of interventions seeking to write disability out of individual and collective futures (Clare 2017; Dolmage 2018; Kafer 2013). Far from being an anomaly, discriminatory triage policies reflect the kind of systemic ableism experienced daily by disabled people in healthcare systems. The adoption of these triage policies only served to amplify existing feel-ings of distrust toward healthcare institutions within the disabled community that are rooted in past and present evidence of institutional neglect and mistreatment. The untrustworthiness of these institutions for disabled people is not a recent phenomenon.

In general, we try to avoid, or at the very least minimize, interactions with untrustworthy individuals once we establish that they are untrustworthy. This can be manageable when the untrustworthy party is a family member we see once a year, an ex-partner whose number we've blocked from our phone, or even a colleague from a different department. Avoiding untrustworthy public institutions presents its own set of challenges given that we rely on these institutions to meet some of our most basic needs. Oppressed and marginalized people are often forced to rely on institutions that have harmed them or members of their communities in the past. Hale Demir-Doğuoğlu and Carolyn McLeod (forthcoming) offer the example of an Indigenous person in Canada who must rely on a general practitioner to provide them with care that is free of discrimination, all the while knowing that Indigenous people have historically been subjected to systemic forms of racism and mistreatment when seeking medical care in Canada. Similarly, disabled people often have no choice but to rely on healthcare institutions they do not trust. Forced reliance should not be equated with restored trust. Institutions must make efforts to repair relations of trust even if socially marginalized groups refuse to rely on them once the presence of more trustworthy alternatives makes such a refusal possible. The next section considers how institutions can begin to repair damaged trust with the disabled community and work to signal their trustworthiness in the future.

Recommendations for Building Institutional Trustworthiness

Being trustworthy comes with a responsibility for signaling one's trustworthiness. If I tell you that I am trustworthy without offering assurances of my trustworthiness, it is unclear whether I am in fact trustworthy. Jones offers the notion of *rich trustworthiness* to describe the work of signaling one's trustworthiness in relation to a particular domain so that others can "work out where—and where not—to turn" to address needs and situations of dependency (2012, 74). I take this to mean, in part, that being trustworthy is an active responsibility that must be translated in concrete deeds. To be trustworthy in a rich sense, a person or institution must demonstrate how and why they are, as well as specify the domains in which they can be counted on. The work of signaling one's trustworthiness is particularly important when trustworthiness must be rebuilt. In what follows, I offer four potential areas of work for medical and public health institutions that wish to cultivate and demonstrate trustworthiness in times of crisis and beyond them. The following recommendations are by no means exhaustive. They are, however, central to the work of acknowledging barriers to trust with marginalized communities and cultivating institutional trustworthiness.

The first step is to acknowledge contemporary institutional mistrust as rooted in ongoing abuse and discrimination against oppressed and marginalized persons. This type of contextualization helps shift our focus toward the issue of institutional *un*-trustworthiness and frame the need for interventions at a collective, rather than individual, level. While this step may seem redundant or merely performative, it is doubtful that relations of trust between a community and its institutions can begin to be repaired without a proper acknowledgment of the grounds for distrust that extends beyond consideration of the present moment. In their reflection on systemic racism during COVID-19, Best et al. (2021) similarly submit that "admitting untrustworthy actions (both committed and omitted) […] and acknowledging that institutional distrust is justifiable" for oppressed communities is a necessary first step to redressing relations of trust (94). As the authors emphasize, however, this step "only starts a process toward reconciliation" (94). It is very possible for violations of trust to be recognized without this leading to any concrete changes in the lives of those who have been harmed by institutional untrustworthiness. The authors offer the case of Michigan's ongoing Flint Water Crisis as an example. Despite official apologies having been issued, the people of Flint are still without access to safe water at a time when sanitary practices like handwashing are recommended to prevent the spread of the virus. In her response to Walensky's remarks about disabled deaths, Wong points out that a mere apology "does not minimize the harm and mistrust" generated by ableist institutional responses to the pandemic (2022). Offering proofs of institutional trustworthiness begins with the task of recognizing past and ongoing failures, but it cannot end here.

Second, medical and public health institutions must adopt an intersectional lens of analysis to consider the differentiated impacts of public health crises on those who are most marginalized in society. To be sure, disability discrimination *is* a major issue with the development of triage policies during COVID-19, and it should be recognized as such. However, our understanding of the responsibilities of public health and medical institutions during this pandemic must also factor how disability is distributed along classed, racial, and gendered lines and how institutional failures both perpetuate and invisibilize the disablement of Black, brown, Indigenous, incarcerated, gender non-conforming, and poor people. Assurances of trustworthiness directed only at those people who fit dominant social understandings of who counts as disabled (e.g., white, cisgender, middle-class citizens of the United States with a legally documented disability) should be treated with suspicion. Hierarchies of deservingness based on class, race, size, gender, or nationality are irreconcilable with just and trustworthy institutions. Institutions must consider the needs and realities of those most impacted by conditions of injustice, whether they fit dominant understandings of disability or not. Where disabled people need concrete assurances that medical and public health institutions can be counted on during a pandemic, Black, Latinx, Indigenous, trans, queer, poor, and fat disabled people and disabled people of color need assurances that racism, cissexism, classism, fatphobia, and other forms of discrimination will not result in their lives being devalued or their needs overlooked.

An example helps illuminate why developing institutional trustworthiness in part depends on adopting an intersectional lens of analysis and intervention. Black disabled people are multiply impacted by health inequities and discrimination during COVID-19. As much research has reported, Black communities have experienced significantly higher rates of infection, hospitalization, and death than white communities (Reyes 2020). Systemic barriers to access to care, testing, and medical resources disproportionately impact Black and Latinx neighborhoods (Lawrence et al., 2021). Furthermore, rates of infection and transmission in jails and prisons, where Black people are incarcerated at five times the rate of their white counterparts, have been alarmingly high throughout the pandemic, much to the indifference of public health and government officials (Merelli 2022). Incarcerated people present higher rates of chronic health conditions than the general population, both because they largely represent sections of the population impacted by adverse health determinants and because incarcerated people are systematically disabled and made ill by conditions of incarceration (Ben-Moshe et al. 2014; Nowotny et al. 2017; Schnittker and John 2007; Schnittker et al. 2011). Daniel Young (2020) reports that "[long] histories of systemic racism, marginalization, and underfunding of community-based treatments have disproportionately filled [American] prisons with Black people with disabilities." Despite these concerning and well-documented observations, the intersection of disability and race has often been overlooked during this crisis. Young explains that "even where COVID data has been stratified, it has been either by race *or* by disability. Almost nothing looks at both race *and* disability" (2020). Crucial data is missing that could help us develop responses to the crisis that better consider its impacts on Black disabled people and other people with intersectional identities. As a result of this oversight, the experiences (and deaths) of multiply marginalized people risk being erased. The fact that public health institutions did not systemically gather non-stratified data on race and disability reflects a poor understanding of how systemic racism and ableism affect the lives of Black disabled people and disabled people of color. It also raises doubts about the ability of these institutions to *recognize* overlapping forms of socially constructed dependency and to *respond* to them adequately, both of which are key markers of trustworthiness.

Thirdly, I suggest that increased clarity about the implicit norms and values driving public health policy and medical practice can bolster institutional trustworthiness. We can better assess the trustworthiness of an institution if we are able to clearly identify the values and principles that guide its decision-making practices and evaluate how and whether they translate into practice. Havi Carel and Ian James Kidd (2021) offer the term institutional opacity to describe "a general tendency within large-scale and internally complex institutions to increasingly become resistant to forms of assessment and understanding" (481). Carel and Kidd remark that some "degree of opacity is unavoidable" (486). The inner workings of a large university hospital, for example, are highly complex and knowledge of them is distributed across institutional actors, departments, and sectors. Yet *too much* opacity can make it difficult for users to understand the basic workings of institutions and feel that they can maintain some level of epistemic agency within them. The authors explain: "When one experiences an institution as opaque, one sees that institution's decisions as strange, its practices obscure, and its reasoning impenetrable" (483). As a result, users navigating an opaque institution may feel alienated when seeking medical care for a loved one, making difficult decisions about a course of treatment, or attempting to make sense of care allocation policies in crisis times. Institutional opacity can erode the public's perception of the trustworthiness of an institution.

Values and norms inform many of our personal decisions; it stands to reason that they would also impact how large institutions navigate difficult choices. Value-ladenness is not *itself* the problem. Issues arise, instead, when it is masked under the cover of neutrality. This makes it difficult to understand where institutions stand in terms of their core commitments. It also makes it difficult to develop alternative suggestions about how these institutions might function in the future, what alternative interests they might defend, and how they can be transformed. As Anita Ho (2011) observes in her discussion of diagnostic and therapeutic practices around disability, problems arise when we downplay "the personal and sociopolitical nature and impact" of diagnoses and clinical recommendations and couch them instead "in [a language] that presumes value-neutrality and objectivity" (110). Over time, value-laden medical evaluations that are "disguised as scientifically objective," and particularly ones that perpetuate certain forms of discrimination, can also become difficult to track and critique (111). This process too can contribute to institutional opacity.

Disability critics have shown that purportedly 'neutral' or 'objective' triage protocols can in fact further discrimination against disabled people based on assumptions about what types of bodies and minds are deemed 'healthy' or 'normal.' More generally, an abundant literature demonstrates how ableist conceptions of human form, appearance, function, and behavior shape medical views about disability (Clare 2017; Hall 2021; Kafer 2011; Reynolds 2018). The ideology of ableism consistently values ability over disability and frames disability as an undesirable or tragic state of being. Given that they often operate at a sub-conscious level, ableist assumptions most often go unexamined. They will not be magically neutralized when comes the time to devise guidance on critical care and resource allocation, especially not when decision-makers are overwhelmed by emotionally and physically exhausting demands on their time and attention. More pointedly, the responsibility for identifying these assumptions must not rest solely on the shoulders of individual healthcare providers. Institutions must ensure that there are mechanisms in place to provide decision-makers with clear guidance about how to prevent discrimination. In June 2020, the California Department of Public Health adopted revised crisis care guidelines after advocacy organizations criticized earlier guidelines for discriminating against fat and disabled people, people of color, and older adults. The revised guidelines explicitly prohibit discrimination on the basis of a range of factors, including race and ethnicity, disability, weight-related disabilities and medical conditions, weight and size, perceived self-worth, perceived quality of life, incarceration status, homelessness, and past or future use of resources (cf. Disability Rights Education and Defense Fund 2020). The guidelines include a directive to appoint a Disability Accommodations Specialist or ombudsperson tasked with ensuring that disabled patients have access to needed accommodations at all times. The guidelines also include pre-emptive recommendations for avoiding or limiting the need for rationing, triage scoring policies that account for pre-existing disabilities, and imposed limitations on the range of conditions that can be considered when evaluating a patient's project length of life. The revised California guidelines were developed in consultation with disability organizations like the Disability Rights Education and Defense Fund, Justice in Aging, Disability Rights California, the #NoBodyIsDisposable Coalition, and Independent Living Resource Center San Francisco. Collaborating with disability organizations on the ground, appointing disabled people to hospital triage policies and including disabled doctors, public health experts, bioethicists, and activists in conversations about pandemic preparedness and response is beneficial for multiple reasons. These strategies can help us better consider the implications of medical and public health practices on disabled people, identify harmful assumptions about disability at play in existing policies, and devise institutional values for a world to come that does not devalue disabled life.

This brings me to my final recommendation. Institutions must harness local expertise and knowledge from disabled people themselves. Cultivating trustworthiness requires that institutions start truly listening to and learning from disabled people. Too often, this happens after a crisis has passed or when mistakes have been made. Dr. Walensky met with representatives from disability organizations only *after* her televised remarks made headlines. While the CDC has committed to consulting with disability groups and advocates moving forward, much remains to be done to mobilize the expertise of disabled people within public health and medical practice. When those whose lives are devalued by ableist, racist, classist, transphobic, and fatphobic systems of oppression are left out of discussions about who gets to live and receive care and who does not, they continue to be put "at the bottom of the list." (Wong 2020) Marina Tsaplina and Joseph A. Stramondo (2021) suggest that recognizing disabled people as moral equals requires practical changes in how triage decisions as made. The authors offer concrete strategies for including disabled people on triage committees (e.g., holding meetings on Zoom to allow disabled committee members to participate while sheltering in place). On a different timescale, educating medical providers about ableist biases in medicine (e.g., by including scholarship by disabled people in the medical education curriculum) can strengthen the trustworthiness of individual providers and that of institutions.

Disabled people also have a wealth of knowledge to contribute about how to survive a global health crisis without leaving the most vulnerable people behind. As disability activist and writer Leah Lakshmi Piepzna-Samarasinha (2021) writes, "like every kind of oppressed people, disabled people are geniuses of staying alive despite everything." When they could not trust institutions and governments to keep them safe during the COVID-19 pandemic, disabled people developed networks of care, support, and information to protect themselves and their communities. Collaborative guides created on-the-fly by sick, elder, fat, and disabled people shared advice about where to seek medical care, patient rights in medical settings, low-cost foods to stock up on, how to disinfect mobility aids, recipes for fragrance free homemade hand sanitizer, or minimizing power use on medical devices (Piepzna-Samarasinha 2020; Fat Rose 2020). These and similar disabled mutual aid initiatives reflect the resourcefulness of disabled people and the wealth of skills and knowledge that keep disabled communities afloat. Although mutual aid work generally unfolds outside of dominant medical and public health institutions for good reason—notably, because these institutions have proved untrustworthy in the past— building bridges with disabled communities and foregrounding the contributions of disabled people must become a priority if institutions wish to develop their own trustworthiness.

Conclusion

The strategies I have identified will no doubt require large-scale efforts from institutions. These strategies challenge both the place typically given to disabled people in society and established epistemic hierarchies which work to preserve the expertise of the few against the knowledge of those with lived experiences of disability. Yet this type of challenge to current institutional structures and modes of functioning is necessary. The COVID-19 pandemic has highlighted the devastating implications of institutional untrustworthiness on oppressed communities and the necessity of building relations of trust based on the recognition of the harms produced by systemic injustice. Building trustworthiness requires time and consistent work. The legacy of past and present institutional failures weighs heavily on the lives of marginalized people and relations of trust can only begin to be repaired if institutions take on this work. Much as the pandemic radically altered social practices and generated previously unimagined scales of grief, it also shed light on what was already there: a world structured by injustices that circumscribe relations of trust.

Notes

1 Instead of distinguishing in this manner between trust and reliance, some scholars argue that what is needed is instead a distinction between types of trust: a predictive sense, that is more akin to reliance, and a normative sense that is closer to what I and other scholars mean by trust. For a helpful overview of this question, see Dormandy (2019).
2 Brennan (2024) investigates this question at length in his excellent essay on the costs and burdens of distrust for people living under conditions of oppression.

Work Cited

Baier, Annette. 1986. "Trust and Antitrust." *Ethics* 96 (2): 231–260.
Barnes, Elizabeth. 2016. *The Minority Body: A Theory of Disability*. Oxford: Oxford University Press.
Ben-Moshe, Liat, Allison C Carey, and Chris Chapman. 2014. *Disability Incarcerated: Imprisonment and Disability in the United States and Canada*. Palgrave Macmillan.
Best, Alicia L., Faith E. Fletcher, Mika Kadono, and Rueben C. Warren. 2021. "Institutional Distrust among African Americans and Building Trustworthiness in the COVID-19 Response: Implications for Ethical Public Health Practice." *Journal of Health Care for the Poor and Underserved* 32 (1): 90–98. https://doi.org/10.1353/hpu.2021.0010
Brennan, Johnny. 2024. "Skepticism, The Virtue of Preemptive Distrust." *The Journal of the American Philosophical Association* 10 (2): 1–18.

Butler, Judith. 2004. *Precarious Life: The Powers of Mourning and Violence*. New York: Verso.

Campbell, Stephen M., and Joseph A. Stramondo. 2017. "The Complicated Relationship of Disability and Well-Being." *Kennedy Institute of Ethics Journal* 27 (2): 151–184. https://doi.org/10.1353/ken.2017.0014

Carel, Havi, and Ian James Kidd. 2021. "Institutional Opacity, Epistemic Vulnerability, and Institutional Testimonial Justice." *International Journal of Philosophical Studies* 29 (4): 473–496. https://doi.org/10.1080/09672559.2021.1997393

Clare, Eli. 2017. *Brilliant Imperfection: Grappling with Cure*. Durham: Duke University Press.

Dembosky, April. 2021. "It's Not Tuskegee. Current Medical Racism Fuels Black Americans' Vaccine Hesitancy." *Los Angeles Times*, March 25, 2021. https://www.latimes.com/science/story/2021-03-25/current-medical-racism-not-tuskegee-expls-vaccine-hesitancy-among-black-americans

Disability Rights Education and Defense Fund. 2020. "Summary of California's Revised Crisis Care Guidelines." *DREDF* June 2020. https://dredf.org/2020/06/10/summary-of-californias-revised-crisis-care-guidelines/

Demir-Doğuoğlu, Hale and Carolyn McLeod. Forthcoming. "Toward a Feminist Theory of Distrust." In *The Moral Psychology of Trust*, edited by D. Collins, M. Alfano and I.V. Javonovic. Lexington Books.

Dolmage, Jay. 2018. *Disabled upon Arrival: Eugenics, Immigration, and the Construction of Race and Disability*. Columbus, OH: Ohio State University Press.

Dormandy, Katherine. 2019. "Introduction: An Overview of Trust and Some Key Epistemological Implications." In *Trust in Epistemology*, edited by Katherine Dormandy, 1–40. New York: Routledge.

Fat Rose. 2020. "Fat-Assed Prepper Survival Tips for Preparing for a Coronavirus Quarantine." *Google Document*, March 12, 2020. https://docs.google.com/document/d/1Zz7EchIvq05wFDZ1EysJkGiMJTpzXxi998M2Ij2hYhg/edit#

Felt, Ashley Brooke, Dionne Mitcham, Morgan Hathcock, Raymond Swienton, and Curtis Harris. 2021. "Discrimination and Bias in State Triage Protocols Toward Populations with Intellectual Disabilities During the COVID-19 Pandemic." *Disaster Medicine and Public Health Preparedness* 16 (5): 1–3. https://doi.org/10.1017/dmp.2021.81

Govier, Trudy. 1992. "Distrust as a Practical Problem." *Journal of Social Philosophy* 23 (1): 52–63.

Gleason, Jonathan, Wendy Ross, Alexander Fossi, Heather Blonsky, Jane Tobias, and Mary Stephens. 2021. "The Devastating Impact of COVID-19 on Individuals with Intellectual Disabilities in the United States." *NEJM Catalyst Innovations in Care Delivery* 2 (2). https://doi.org/10.1056/CAT.21.0051

Hall, Kim Q. 2021. "Limping Along: Toward a Crip Phenomenology." *The Journal of Philosophy of Disability* 1: 11–33. https://doi.org/10.5840/jpd20218275

Hansford, Rebecca, Hélène Ouellette-Kuntz, and Lynn Martin. 2022. "Short Report: The Influence of Congregate Setting on Positive COVID-19 Tests among a High-Risk Sample of Adults with Intellectual and Developmental Disability in Ontario." *Research in Developmental Disabilities* 122: 104178. https://doi.org/10.1016/j.ridd.2022.104178

Ho, Anita. 2011. "Trusting Experts and Epistemic Humility in Disability." *International Journal of Feminist Approaches to Bioethics* 4 (2): 102–23. https://doi.org/10.2979/intjfemappbio.4.2.102

Iezzoni, Lisa I., Sowmya R. Rao, Julie Ressalam, Dragana Bolcic-Jankovic, Nicole D. Agaronnik, Karen Donelan, Tara Lagu, and Eric G. Campbell. 2021. "Physicians' Perceptions of People with Disability and Their Health Care." *Health Affairs* 40 (2): 297–306. https://doi.org/10.1377/hlthaff.2020.01452

Jones, Karen. 2004. "Trust and Terror." In *Moral Psychology: Feminist Ethics and Social Theory*, edited by Peggy DesAutels and Margaret Urban Walker, 3–18. Lanham, MD: Rowman & Littlefield.

Jones, Karen. 2012. "Trustworthiness." *Ethics* 123 (1): 61–85.

Kafer, Alison. 2011. "Debating Feminist Futures: Slippery Slopes, Cultural Anxiety, and the Case of the Deaf Lesbians." In *Feminist Disability Studies*, edited by Kim Q. Hall, 218–241. Bloomington, IN: Indiana University Press.

Kafer, Alison. 2013. *Feminist, Queer, Crip*. Bloomington, IN: Indiana University Press.

Kittay, Eva Feder. 1999. *Love's Labor: Essays on Women, Equality and Dependency*. New York: Routledge.

Kothari, Sunil. 2004. "Clinical (Mis) Judgments of Quality of Life After Disability." *Journal of Clinical Ethics* 15 (4): 300–307.

Lawrence, Carissa, Divya Manoharan, Zackary Berger, and Karla F. C. Holloway. 2021. "Vaccine Hesitancy Is No Excuse for Systemic Racism." *The Hastings Center*, February 25, 2021. https://www.thehastingscenter.org/vaccine-hesitancy-is-no-excuse-for-systemic-racism/

Leonard, Mary B., DeWayne M. Pursley, Lisa A. Robinson, Steven H. Abman, and Jonathan M. Davis. 2022. "The Importance of Trustworthiness: Lessons from the COVID-19 Pandemic." *Pediatric Research* 91 (3): 482–485. https://doi.org/10.1038/s41390-021-01866-z

Marcelin, Jasmine R, Talia H Swartz, Fidelia Bernice, Vladimir Berthaud, Robbie Christian, Christopher da Costa, Nada Fadul. 2021. "Addressing and Inspiring Vaccine Confidence in Black, Indigenous, and People of Color During the Coronavirus Disease 2019 Pandemic." *Open Forum Infectious Diseases* 8 (9): ofab417. https://doi.org/10.1093/ofid/ofab417

Mello, Michelle M., Govind Persad, and Douglas B. White. 2020. "Respecting Disability Rights — Toward Improved Crisis Standards of Care." *New England Journal of Medicine* 383 (5): e26. https://doi.org/10.1056/NEJMp2011997

Merelli, Annalisa. 2022. "The Origins of COVID-19's Racial Disparities Lie in America's Prisons." *Quartz*, June 14, 2021. https://qz.com/2019954/overcrowded-prisons-help-explain-us-covid-19-racial-inequality/

Metzl, Jonathan, and Anna Kirkland. 2010. *Against Health: How Health Became the New Morality.* New York: New York University Press.

Miller, Sarah Clark. 2011. *The Ethics of Need: Agency, Dignity, and Obligation.* New York: Routledge. https://doi.org/10.4324/9780203334393

Mitchell, David T, and Sharon L Snyder. 2015. *The Biopolitics of Disability: Neoliberalism, Ablenationalism, and Peripheral Embodiment.* Ann Arbor: University of Michigan Press, 2015.

Mollow, Anna. 2017. "Unvictimizable: Toward a Fat Black Disability Studies." *African American Review* 50 (2): 105–121.

U.N. Department of Economic and Social Affairs. "Five Things You Need to Know about Living with a Disability during COVID-19." *United Nations.* https://www.un.org/en/desa/five-things-you-need-know-about-living-disability-during-covid-19

Ne'eman, Ari. 2020. "Opinion | 'I Will Not Apologize for My Needs.'" *The New York Times*, March 23, 2020. https://www.nytimes.com/2020/03/23/opinion/coronavirus-ventilators-triage-disability.html

Nowotny, Kathryn M., Richard G. Rogers, and Jason D. Boardman. 2017. "Racial Disparities in Health Conditions among Prisoners Compared with the General Population." *SSM - Population Health* 3: 487–496. https://doi.org/10.1016/j.ssmph.2017.05.011

Pearl, Robert. 2023. "U.S. Healthcare: A Conglomerate of Monopolies." *Forbes*, January 16, 2023. https://www.forbes.com/sites/robertpearl/2023/01/16/us-healthcare-a-conglomerate-of-monopolies/

Piepzna-Samarasinha, Leah Lakshmi. 2020. "Half Assed Disabled Prepper Tips for Preparing for a Coronavirus Quarantine." *Google Documents*, March 9, 2020. https://docs.google.com/document/d/1rIdpKgXeBHbmM3KpB5NfjEBue8YN1MbXhQ7zTOLmSyo/edit

Piepzna-Samarasinha, Leah Lakshmi. 2021. "How Disabled Mutual Aid Is Different Than Abled Mutual Aid." *Disability Visibility Project*, October 3, 2021. https://disabilityvisibilityproject.com/2021/10/03/how-disabled-mutual-aid-is-different-than-abled-mutual-aid/

Potter, Nancy Nyquist. 2002. *How Can I Be Trusted? A Virtue Theory of Trustworthiness.* Lanham, MD: Rowman & Littlefield.

PressProgress. 2021. "Disability Groups Say Ontario Government Did Not Consult Them on Life and Death COVID-19 'Triage' Decisions." *PressProgress*, May 6, 2021. https://pressprogress.ca/disability-groups-say-ontario-government-did-not-consult-them-on-life-and-death-covid-19-triage-decisions/

Quinn, Sandra C., and Michele P. Andrasik. 2021. "Addressing Vaccine Hesitancy in BIPOC Communities — Toward Trustworthiness, Partnership, and Reciprocity." *The New England Journal of Medicine* 385 (2): 97–100. https://doi.org/10.1056/NEJMp2103104

Reynolds, Joel Michael. 2022 *The Life Worth Living: Disability, Pain, and Morality.* Minneapolis, MN: University of Minnesota Press.

Reynolds, Joel Michael. 2018. "Three Things Clinicians Should Know About Disability." *AMA Journal of Ethics* 20 (12): 1181–1187. https://doi.org/10.1001/amajethics.2018.1181

Reynolds, Joel Michael, Laura Guidry-Grimes, and Katie Savin. 2021. "Against Personal Ventilator Reallocation." *Cambridge Quarterly of Healthcare Ethics* 30 (2): 1–13. https://doi.org/10.1017/S0963180120000833

Rogers, Wendy, Catriona Mackenzie, and Susan Dodds. 2012. "Why Bioethics Needs a Concept of Vulnerability." *International Journal of Feminist Approaches to Bioethics* 5 (2): 11–38. https://doi.org/10.2979/intjfemappbio.5.2.11

Rosalsky, Greg. 2021. "The Untamed Rise of Hospital Monopolies." *National Public Radio*, July 20, 2021. https://www.npr.org/sections/money/2021/07/20/1017631111/the-untamed-rise-of-hospital-monopolies

Schnittker, Jason, and Andrea John. 2007. "Enduring Stigma: The Long-Term Effects of Incarceration on Health." *Journal of Health and Social Behavior* 48 (2): 115–130. https://doi.org/10.1177/002214650704800202

Schnittker, Jason, Michael Massoglia, and Christopher Uggen. 2011. "Incarceration and the health of the African American Community." *Du Bois Review: Social Science Research on Race* 8 (1): 133–141. https://doi.org/10.1017/S1742058X11000026

Scully, Jackie Leach. 2020. "Disability, Disablism, and COVID-19 Pandemic Triage." *Journal of Bioethical Inquiry* 17 (4): 601–605. https://doi.org/10.1007/s11673-020-10005-y

Solomon, Mildred Z., Matthew K. Wynia, and Lawrence O. Gostin. 2020. "COVID-19 Crisis Triage — Optimizing Health Outcomes and Disability Rights." *The New England Journal of Medicine* 383 (5): e27. https://doi.org/10.1056/NEJMp2008300

Stramondo, Joseph. 2020. "COVID-19 Triage and Disability: What NOT To Do." *Bioethics Today*, March 30, 2020. https://bioethicstoday.org/blog/covid-19-triage-and-disability-what-not-to-do/

Stramondo, Joseph A. 2021. "Bioethics, Adaptive Preferences, and Judging the Quality of a Life with Disability." *Social Theory and Practice* 47 (1): 199–220. https://doi.org/10.5840/soctheorpract202121117

Gilson, Erin. 2013. *The Ethics of Vulnerability: A Feminist Analysis of Social Life and Practice*. New York: Routledge.

Tremain, Shelley. 2020. "COVID-19 and The Naturalization of Vulnerability." *Biopolitical Philosophy*, April 1, 2020. https://biopoliticalphilosophy.com/2020/04/01/covid-19-and-the-naturalization-of-vulnerability/

Tsaplina, Marina, and Joseph A. Stramondo. 2020. "#WeAreEssential: Why Disabled People Should Be Appointed to Hospital Triage Committees." *The Hastings Center*, May 15, 2020. https://www.thehastingscenter.org/weareessential-why-disabled-people-should-be-appointed-to-hospital-triage-committees/

Vasquez Reyes, Maritza. 2020. "The Disproportional Impact of COVID-19 on African Americans." *Health and Human Rights* 22 (2): 299–307.

Warren, Rueben C., Lachlan Forrow, David Augustin Hodge, and Robert D. Truog. 2020. "Trustworthiness before Trust—COVID-19 Vaccine Trials and the Black Community." *New England Journal of Medicine* 383 (22): e121.

What We Don't Understand about Trust, n.d. 1380121621. https://www.ted.com/talks/onora_o_neill_what_we_don_t_understand_about_trust

O'Neill, Onora. 2013. "What We Don't Understand About Trust." Filmed June 2013 at TEDxHousesOfParliament, London, United Kingdom. Video. https://www.ted.com/talks/onora_o_neill_what_we_don_t_understand_about_trust?language=en

Wong, Alice. 2020. "I'm Disabled and Need a Ventilator to Live. Am I Expendable during This Pandemic?" *Vox*, April 4, 2020. https://www.vox.com/first-person/2020/4/4/21204261/coronavirus-covid-19-disabled-people-disabilities-triage

Wong, Alice. 2022. "Twitter Post from January 12, 2022." *Twitter*, January 12, 2022. https://twitter.com/SFdirewolf/status/1481143771215523842?ref_src=twsrc%5Etfw%7Ctwcamp%5Etweetembed%7Ctwterm%5E1481143771215523842%7Ctwgr%5E%7Ctwcon%5Es1_&ref_url=https%3A%2F%2Fcaliforniahealthline.org%2Fnews%2Farticle%2Fa-disabled-activist-speaks-out-about-feeling-disposable%2F

Young, Daniel. 2020. "Black, Disabled, and Uncounted." *National Health Law Program*, August 7, 2020. https://healthlaw.org/black-disabled-and-uncounted/

Zhu, Jane, Connor T. A. Brenna, Liam G. McCoy, Chloë G. K. Atkins, and Sunit Das. 2022. "An Ethical Analysis of Clinical Triage Protocols and Decision-Making Frameworks: What Do the Principles of Justice, Freedom, and a Disability Rights Approach Demand of Us?" *BMC Medical Ethics* 23 (1): 11. https://doi.org/10.1186/s12910-022-00749-0

INDEX

Pages in *italics* refer to figures, pages in **bold** refer to tables, and pages followed by n refer to notes.

ableism 18–19, 35, 124; and COVID-19 pandemic 19, 76–77; within healthcare institutions 36; and racism 78–79
Affordable Care Act (ACA) 38, 154
Americans with Disabilities Act (ADA) 5–6, 11n7, 19, 96, 99, 139, 154
Anderson, Elizabeth 145

bioethics 136; and COVID-19 51–53; and disability justice 4–5

CalFresh benefits 67–68
chronic injustice 71, 73–76
Combahee River Collective 6
COVID-19 1–3, 20, 23, 35, 38, 47, 59, 63–68, 98, 107, 120, 135, 145; COVID-19-related deaths 2, 74, 86, 120, 154; and intellectual disability 99; Omicron variant 117n3, 154; triage protocols *see* triage
crip doulaship 116, 131
Crisis Standards of Care (CSOS): discrimination within 35–37; The Institute of Medicine Committee on Guidance for Establishing Standards of Care for Use in Disaster Situations 33, 37; State of Alabama Emergency Operations Plan 4, **22**, 39, 47, 154
critical disability studies 61–62

disability activism 7, 19, 116; and COVID-19 17, 159; and long COVID 87
disability community 23, 27, 38, 88–89, 91, 129, 154

disability justice 4–7, 19, 79, 91–92, 111–117, 128–131; versus disability rights 19–22, 128; and intersectionality 6, 52–53, 96; lineages of 5; "Ten Principles of Disability Justice" 113–116, 117n4
disability rights 5–6, 19, **22**, 53, 96; as anti-discrimination approach 21; shortcomings of 5, 96

employment discrimination 66–67
Eugenics 17, 28n3, 51, 128

Frye, Marilyn 141–142

healthcare disparities: and COVID-19 77, 111; and disability 18, 22, 34, 36, 95, 97; and race 34, 36, 40, 77, 111, 157

Individuals with Disabilities Education Act (IDEA) 19, 137–140; and private schools 146n4
institutional trustworthiness 150; building trust 156–160; and COVID-19 153–156; and vulnerability 151–152
intellectual disability 95–97, 101, 146n15

Lewis, Talila A 18, 36, 78
Liasidou, Anastasia 137
long Covid 84–85; as disability 85–87; as mass disabling event 109–111; and National Institutes of Health 87, 116
The Long COVID Justice Project 108, 114–116

Michael Hickson case 25
Mingus, Mia 113, 115

National Council on Disability 98
Ne'eman, Ari 23, 47

O'Neill, Onora 150

pandemic preparedness 90–92, 159
patient-centered care 95
Piepzna-Samarasinha, Leah Lakshmi 112–113, 116, 130, 159–160
Puar, Jasbir 72, 80n3, 107–108

quality adjusted life years (QALYs) 98–101

racialized disablement 71, 77–79
Russell, Marta 11n7

Sarah McSweeney case 25
Scully, Jackie Leach 7, 34, 50, 136
Section 8 housing 65
Sequential Organ Failure Assessment (SOFA): and COVID-19 40–41; discrimination within 40; use within crisis standards of care 40–41
Sins Invalid 5, 19, 113–114
social determinants of health (SDH) 33–35

Social Security Disability Income (SSDI): and COVID-19 61; and Federal Poverty Line *60*
Social Security Model of Disability *62*
sociopolitical production of disability 72–73

Tremain, Shelley 51–53
triage 4, 20–21, 24, 34, 42, 98, 154; ableism within **22**, 154–156; Canada's COVID-19 Triage Protocol 154; and COVID-19 17, 24–25, 38–39, 47–49, 100, 157; and disability justice 24–26; triage teams/committees 42, 50, 159

U.S. Department of Health and Human Services 3, 38, 47, 117n1, 124; investigations into triage policies 21, 154

Ventilator reallocation 41

Wills, Vanessa 135
Wong, Alice 5, 154
World Health Organization (WHO) 1, 136; *Public Health Emergency of International Concern (PHEIC)* 1

Young, Iris Marion 142, 146n10, 146n13

Zack, Naomi 2, 11n1, 135

Printed in the United States
by Baker & Taylor Publisher Services